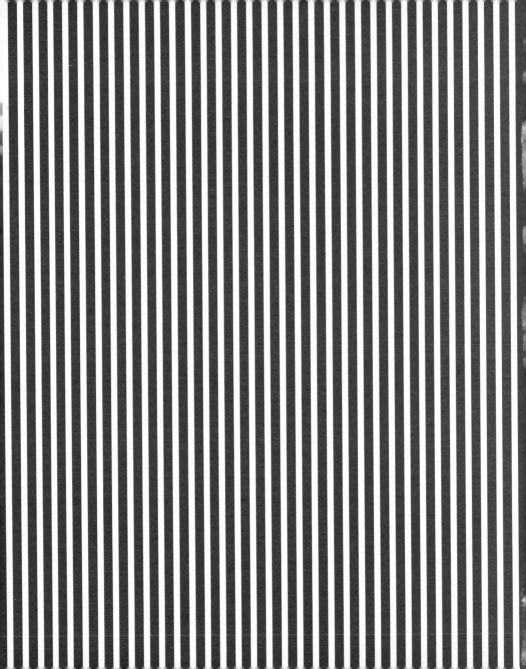

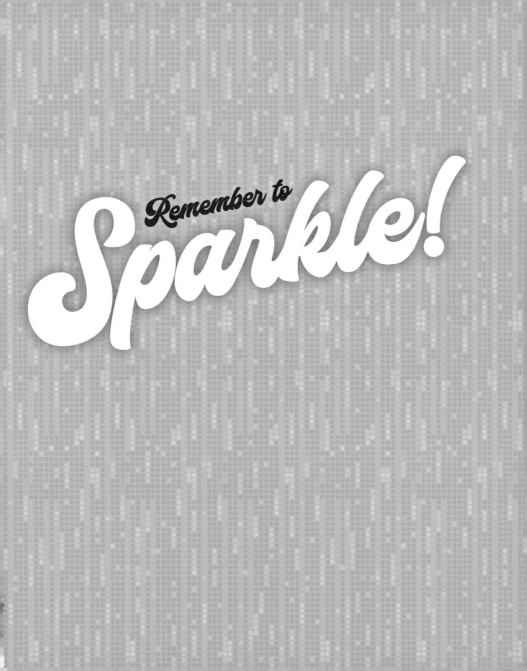

Running Press
Hachette Book Group
1290 Avenue of the Americas, New York, NY 10104
www.runningpress.com
@Running_Press

Printed in China

First Edition: October 2021

Published by Running Press, an imprint of Perseus Books, LLC, a subsidiary of Hachette Book Group, Inc. The Running Press name and logo is a trademark of the Hachette Book Group.

The Hachette Speakers Bureau provides a wide range of authors for speaking events. To find out more, go to www.hachettespeakersbureau.com or call (866) 376-6591.

The publisher is not responsible for websites (or their content) that are not owned by the publisher.

Print book cover and interior design
by Susan Van Horn

Library of Congress Control Number: 2021937577

ISBNs: 978-0-7624-7541-4 (hardcover),
978-0-7624-7539-1 (ebook)

RRD-S

10  9  8  7  6  5  4  3  2  1

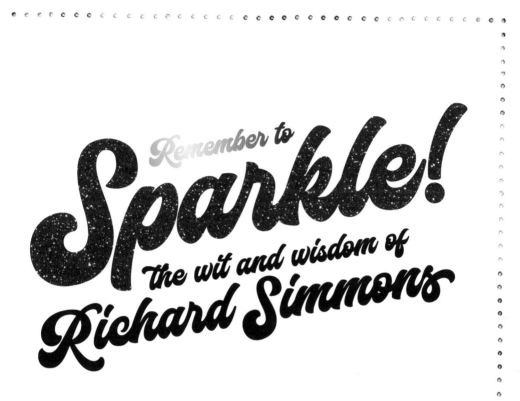

# Remember to Sparkle!

## the wit and wisdom of Richard Simmons

**ROBB PEARLMAN**

RUNNING PRESS

PHILADELPHIA

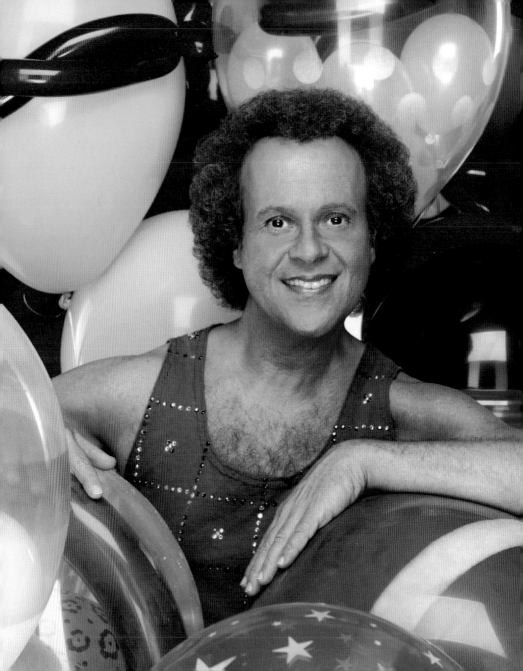

**RICHARD SIMMONS** may be best-known to today's audiences as an enigmatic and elusive sprite with a hairdo as iconic as his wardrobe of short shorts and tank tops. But ask any one of the thousands who have taken his exercise classes, or the countless millions who have met him or seen him in person or on television, and they will tell you that there's so much more to Richard than meets the eye. Richard's words, and the sincerity he put behind them, changed peoples' lives. So it's perhaps those folks who were inspired to take control of their lives who truly understand *who* Richard is, and *what* he believes. He believes that rather than filling your stomach with empty calories, you need to fill your heart with love. He believes that rather than wasting energy with worry or anxiety, you should channel your energy into exercising your body and your spirit. But, most importantly, Richard believes in you.

Whether it was through his exercise classes, television shows, books, *Sweatin' to the Oldies* videos, Deal-a-Meal weight loss program, or even as a headliner on national mall tours or international cruises, Richard's workouts worked out more than muscles; they allowed his fans—his friends—to shed not only pounds, but the emotional baggage that kept them too physically and spiritually weighed down to achieve their goals. Because, at the end of the day—or the class—it wasn't about counting steps, it was about taking the steps to make a better, more fulfilling, and more authentic life.

And the reason millions of fans have been successful over the course of Richard's 40-plus years in the spotlight is not just because Richard believed they could be, but because he helped them believe in their own success, too. They've been able to move their bodies to shed pounds, start new careers, grow their families, and become active, engaged, and joyful participants in their own lives—and in the lives of their family and friends.

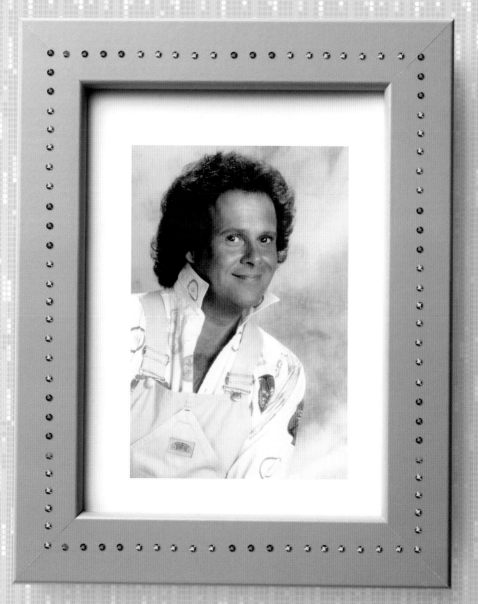

# *Richard's story*

**BEFORE HE ENCOURAGED OTHERS TO SWEAT TO THE OLDIES,** Richard Simmons sweated in the heat and humidity of New Orleans' French Quarter, where he was born to Shirley and Leonard Simmons as Milton Teagle Simmons, and (French) bread on a steady diet of spicy jazz and sweet desserts. By Richard's own account, the Simmons family too often equated food with love, and the ritualization of mealtimes in the household—especially the meticulously planned, multicourse suppers young Milton and his older brother Lenny enjoyed—would rival the elaborate rituals occurring during any religious service. By the time he reached high school, Milton weighed more than 250 pounds and was struggling.

Though the name "Milton" may have been perfect for an accountant, and his weight might have been perfect for a football player, both were ill-suited to the boy's more outgoing and artistic personality. He found himself unable to take full advantage of the active lifestyle enjoyed by most of his peers. And though a portion of his weight was made up of several French Markets' worth of smarts and sass, it was mostly just fat—fat that resulted from a fundamentally dysfunctional relationship with food. He felt stuck. In his city, in his body, and in his mind-set. So, he decided to make some changes.

First was changing his name. He never *felt* like a Milton—whatever a Milton was supposed to feel like—so he decided that he would be called "Richard," after his beloved uncle. His family was supportive of the decision (perhaps in hopes that small changes would lead him to be less argumentative with his father and, maybe, less irreverent) and encouraged him to make other positive changes. Inspired by his friend's mother, Richard decided to try to lose weight by attending local Weight Watchers meetings. But after some time, he found their methods less motivating than they were disheartening, so he quit. Richard came to realize that he wouldn't be able to rely on others to show him a path for success. He would have to look within himself to feel—and be—truly motivated to make the positive changes that would grant him control over his weight, his life, and his destiny.

In 1973, without a job or much of a plan, Richard packed his bags and moved west to Los Angeles to make his own way in the world. He spent his days working in restaurants and his off-hours trying to find a comfortable place to exercise and shed the pounds he had carried with him from New Orleans. Unfortunately, most of the gyms and studios at the time catered to an already-fit clientele and were not particularly welcoming to those whose bodies did not reflect a more traditional physical ideal. It was clear to Richard that overweight people were, in fact, an underserved community, and it reminded him of how he felt—and the lessons he learned—back in New Orleans. He knew he could not look to others, but instead needed to dig deep within himself to be the change he wanted to see in himself, and the world.

In 1974, Richard opened his first exercise studio, the Anatomy

OPPOSITE: Richard leading a class in 1978

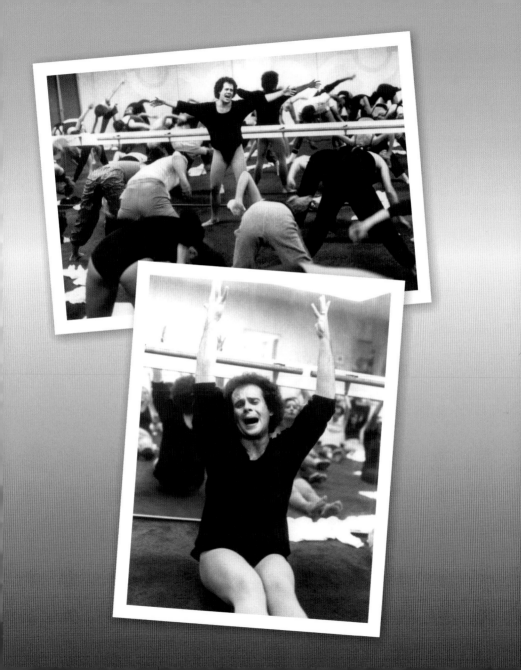

Asylum. Decades before the terms "body positivity" and "safe space" were ever coined, the budding fitness guru was a pioneer in establishing the spirit of those now-ubiquitous phrases. Richard worked with medical professionals to ensure that he offered people of all shapes and sizes, all fitness levels, and all ages, a place where they could feel supported and motivated to exercise their way toward reaching their health and fitness goals. Before long, he changed the studio's name to Slimmons, but the classes he offered remained fun, energetic, and thoughtful. Nobody was ever shamed for not losing weight. Instead, Richard tried to find novel ways to burn calories and keep dieters focused on their goals. He knew that the only true motivation for getting people to make changes in their life was to get them to believe that they were "worth it." Everyone, Richard believed,

RIGHT: Richard with an exercise class in 1983

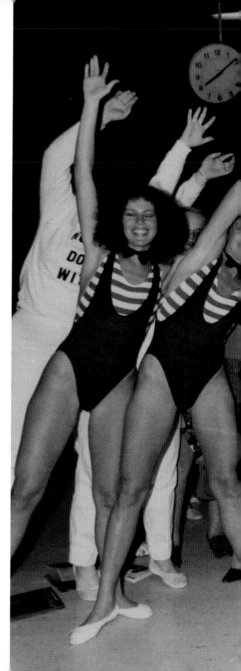

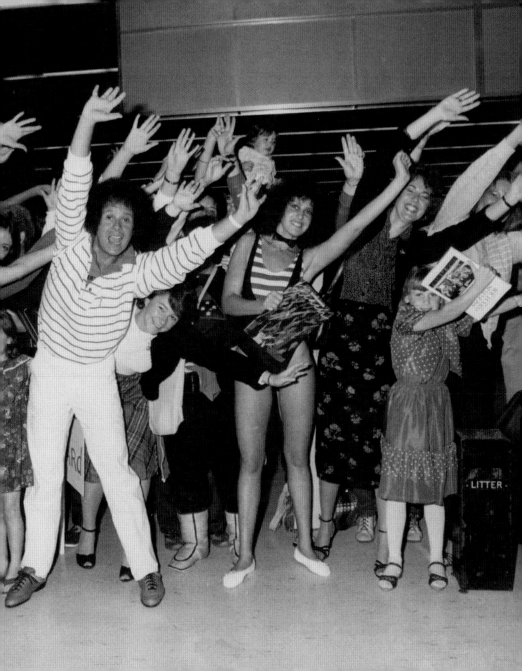

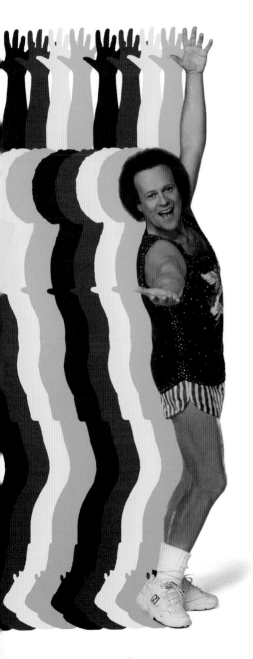

was special, and deserving of as much health, love, and attention as anyone else. With this ethos permeating every class, members became family and friends who provided one another with ongoing emotional support, and, by way of their clear, measurable weight loss, Richard himself saw proof that his methods worked.

Before long, the media took notice of Richard's ethos, incomparable personality, and the remarkable results coming out of his exercise studio. The fitness instructor was soon a featured guest on news and talk programs, and even game shows. Then, in 1980, he got his own television program: *The Richard Simmons Show*. Part talk show, part at-home exercise class, part motivational session, the program gave Richard a platform to expand his reach and share his singular brand of humor, positivity, and exercises with millions of new fans across the world.

Over the years, Richard was able to further expand his reach through additional television and media appearances (including and especially as a headline-making guest on *David Letterman* and other talk shows), nationwide mall tours, a series of successful cruises, a line of videotapes for at-home workouts, calorie-counting programs, and more. Richard was also a pioneer on social media, and actively engaged with his fans via his website and other online platforms. Recognizing that human connection is, perhaps, the greatest gift one can give, Richard logged countless hours calling people who contacted him to make sure they were all right, on track, and know that they have his support.

Though he would certainly attribute any weight loss success to the person who put in the sweat, it's estimated that, over the years, Richard has helped people lose more than three million pounds. But anyone who has been touched by Richard's honest love for his fellow human beings—through their good times and bad—would certainly agree that they would never have been able to achieve their success without his spirit and unparalleled energy supporting them along the way.

It's Richard's determination to make the world a better place that has made him one of the most iconic and best-loved personalities in the world—a force that not only brought love and laughter to untold millions, but also helped to motivate each and every one of those people to make their own positive, life-affirming changes. Like ripples in a pond, Richard Simmons has radiated outward to enlighten, and lighten, the world around him.

This collection of some of Richard's most wise and witty words is intended to continue his life's work.

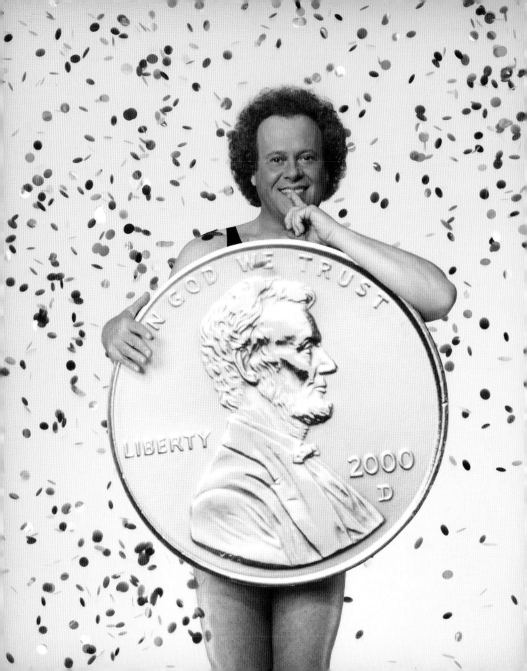

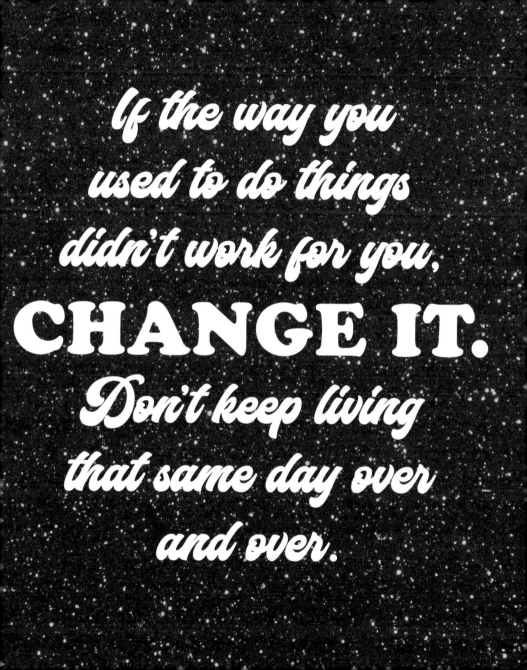

*Forgive yourself*
for the mistakes
you've made, and
*be proud of yourself*
because you're
doing better!

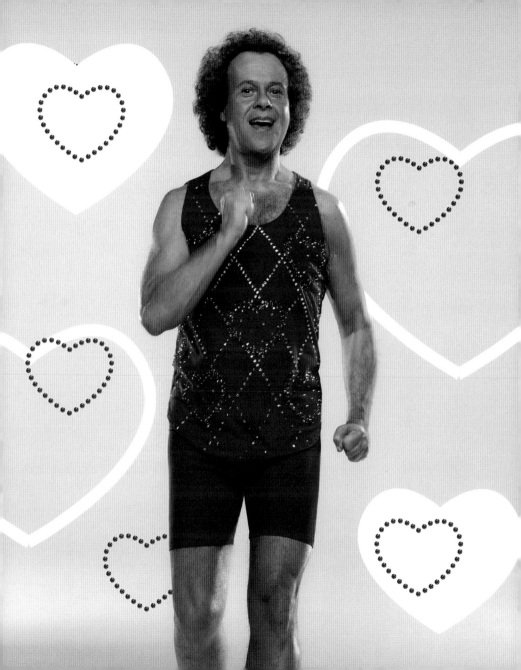

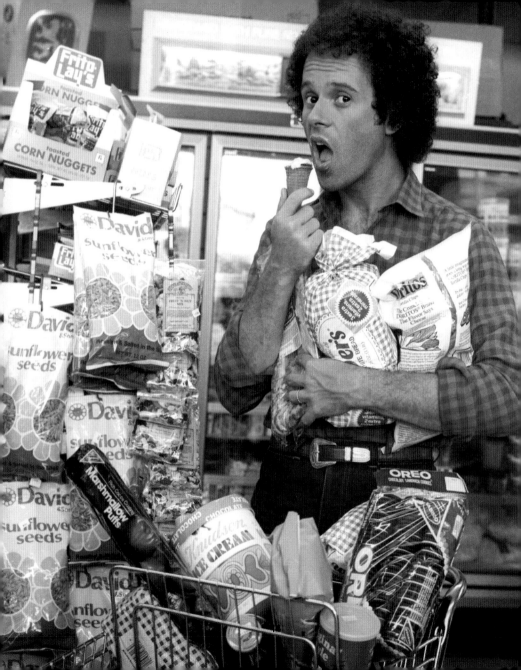

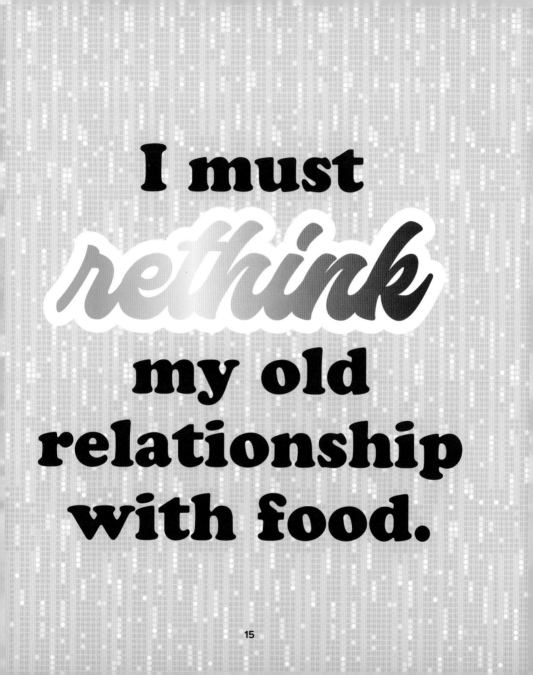

I must *rethink* my old relationship with food.

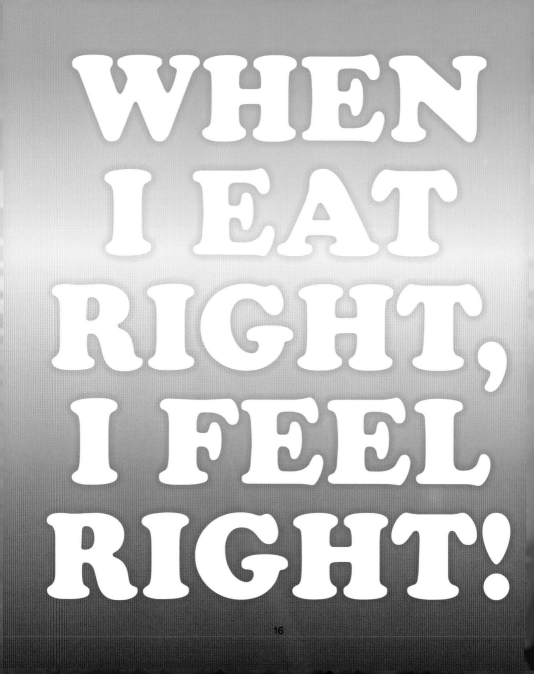

WHEN
I EAT
RIGHT,
I FEEL
RIGHT!

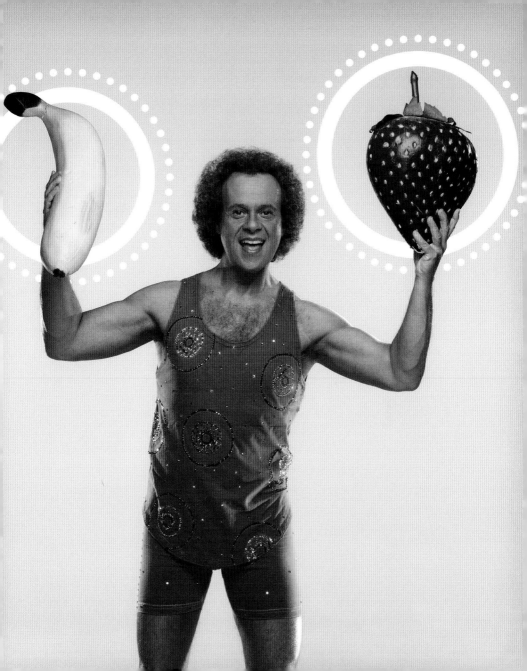

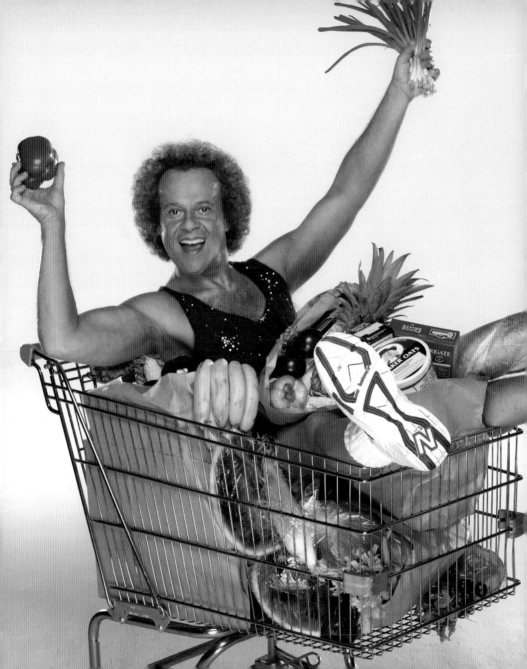

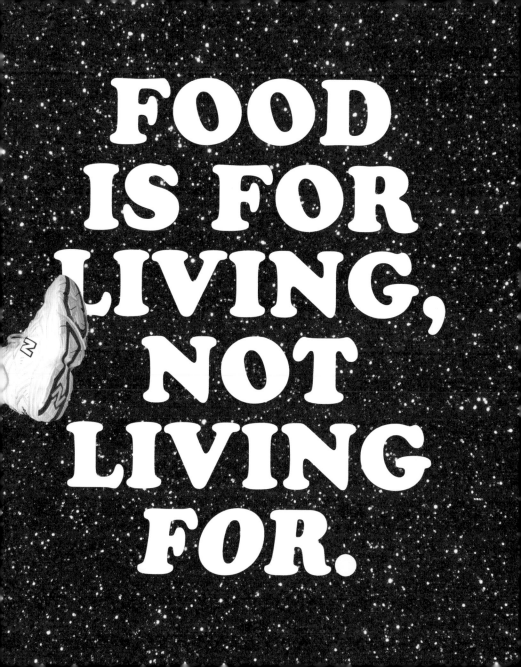

One day at a time, one meal at a time,

*I will take better care of myself!*

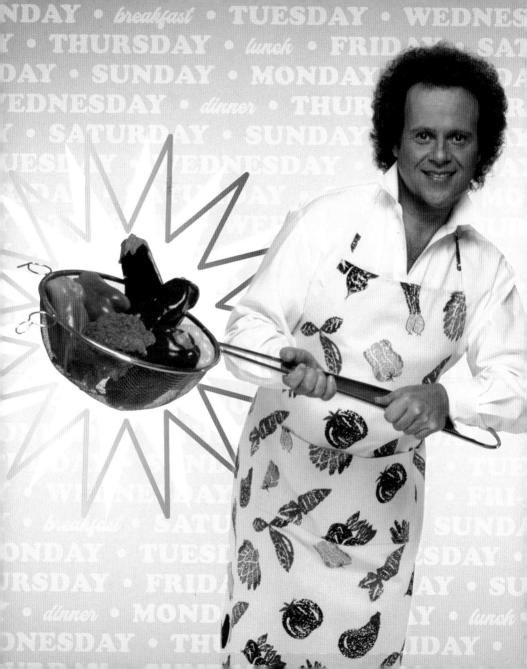

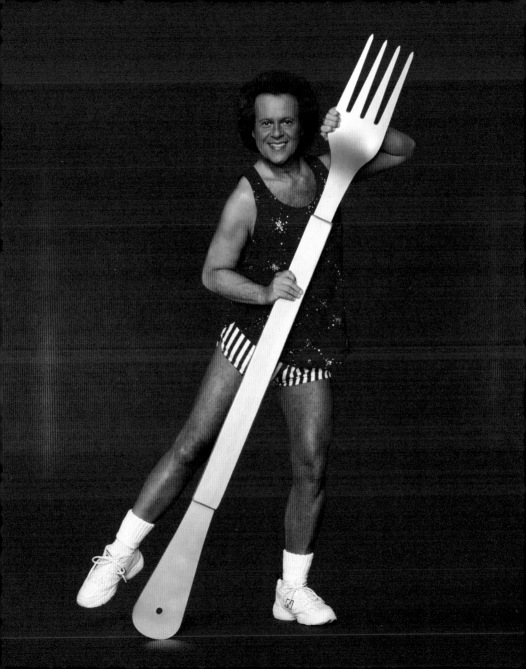

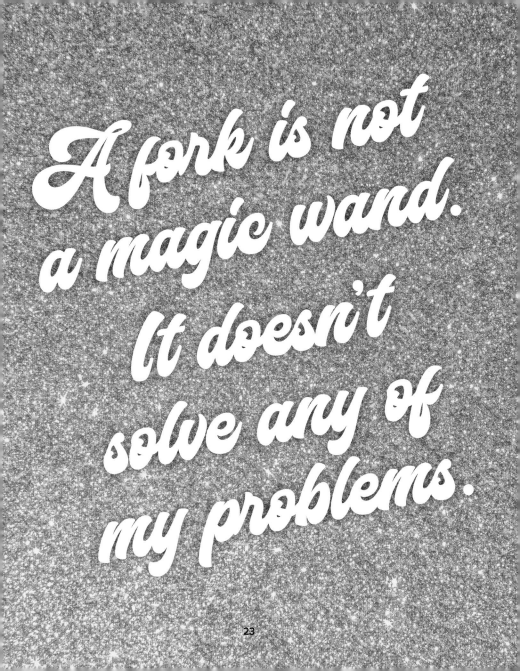

A fork is not a magic wand. It doesn't solve any of my problems.

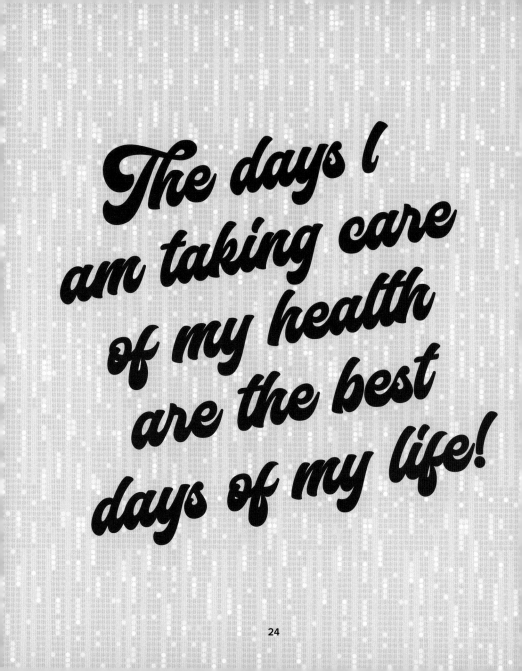

The days I am taking care of my health are the best days of my life!

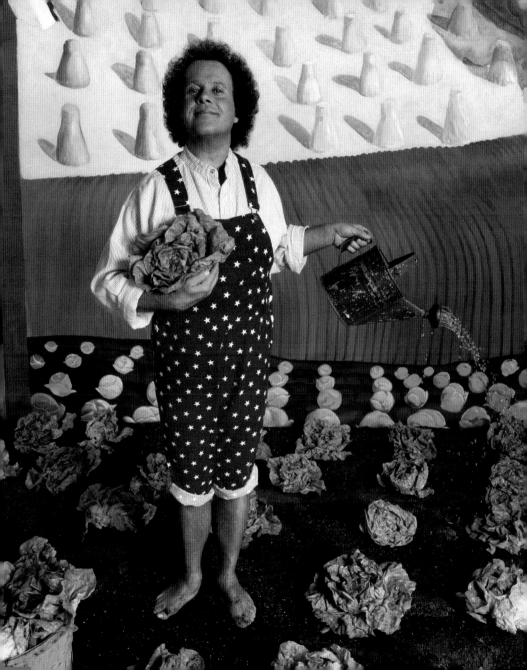

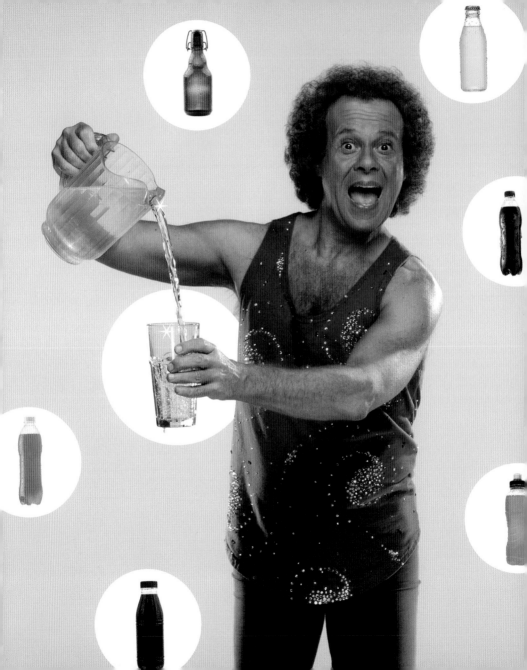

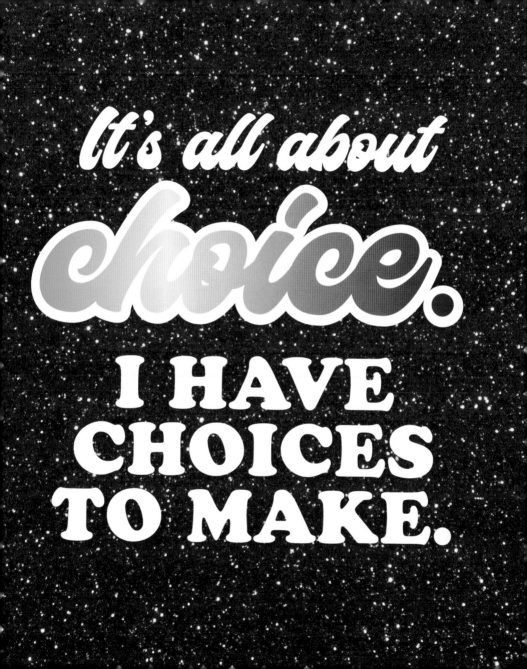

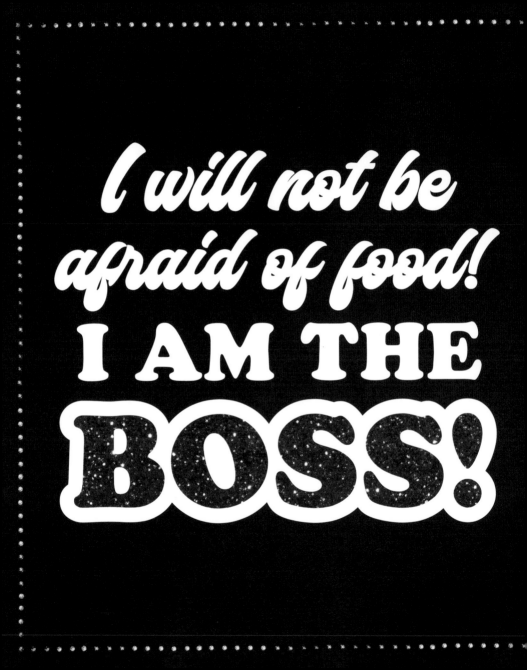

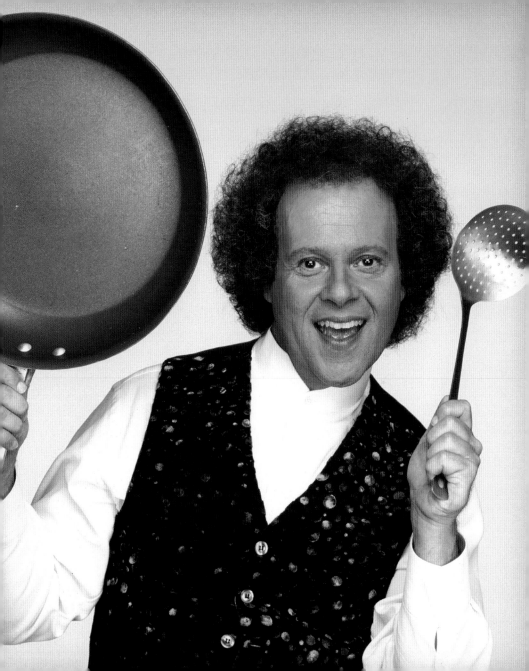

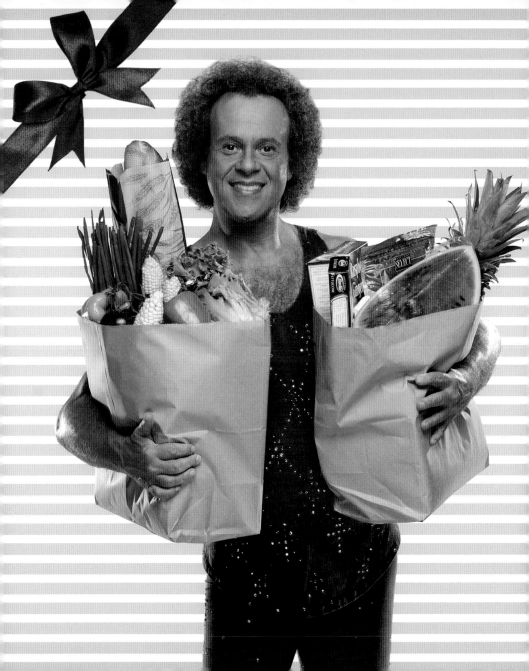

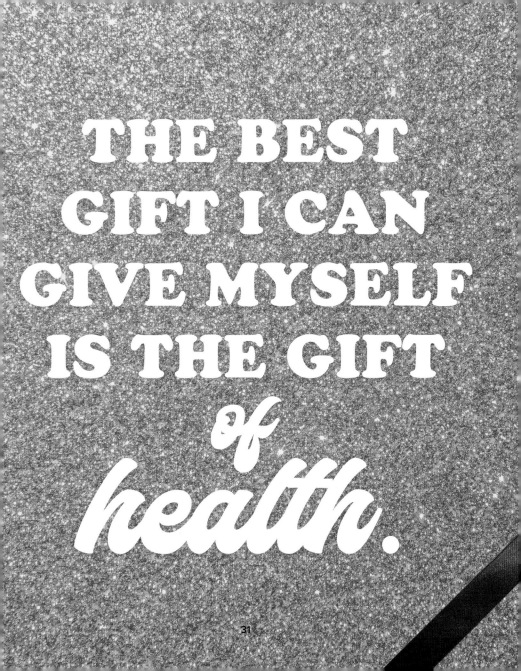

THE BEST
GIFT I CAN
GIVE MYSELF
IS THE GIFT
*of*
*health.*

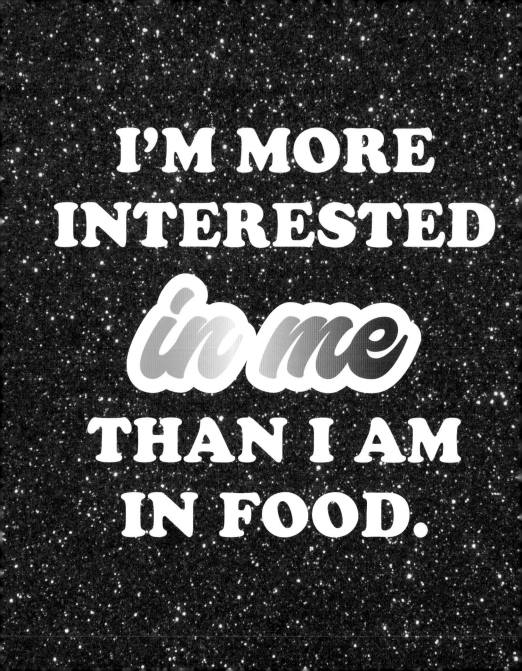

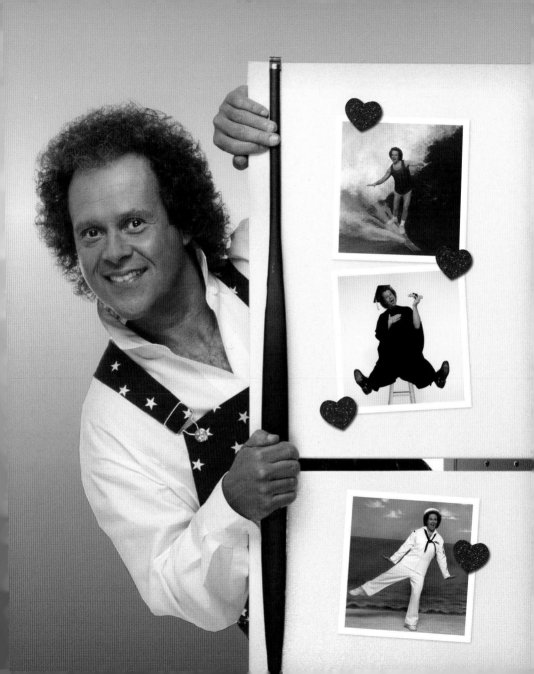

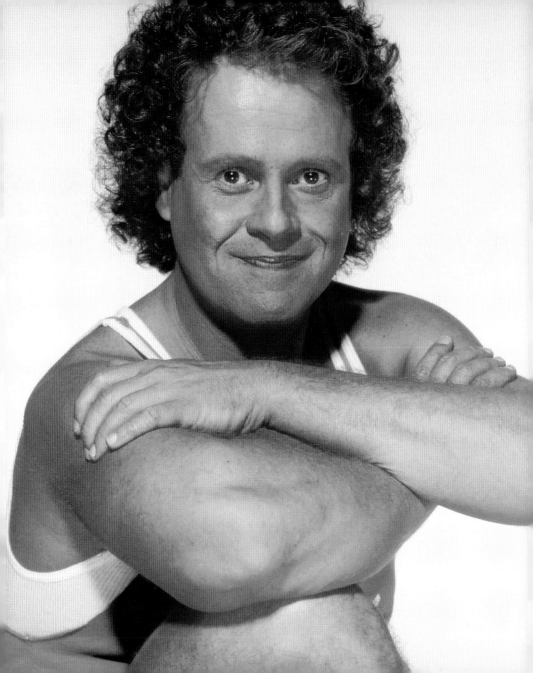

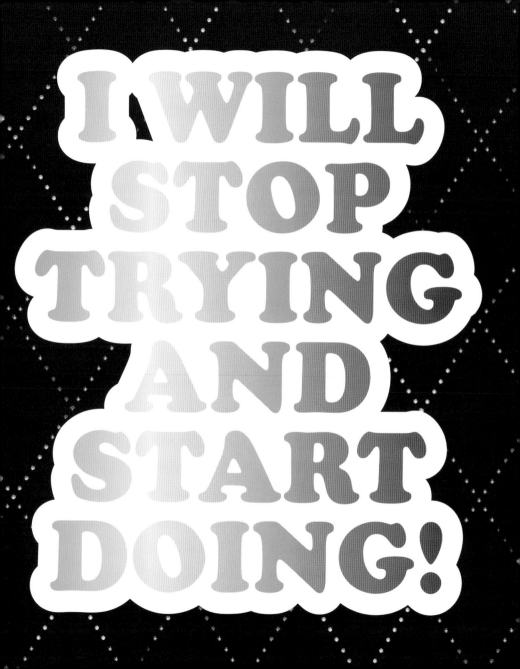

# I WILL MAKE EXERCISE FEEL LIKE MY OWN LITTLE

## party!

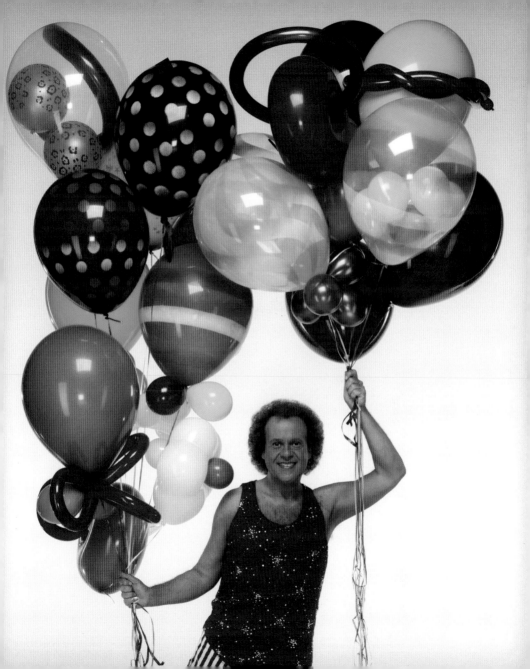

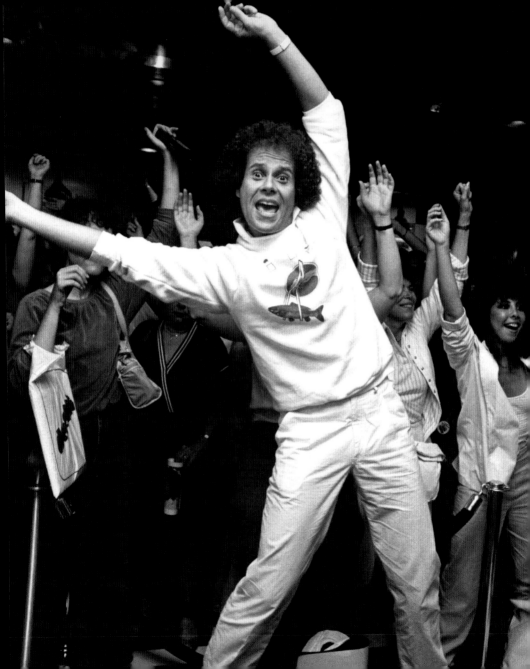

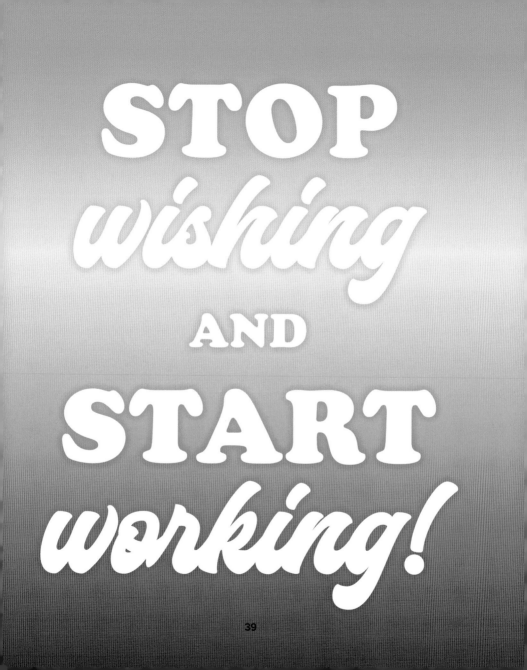

STOP *wishing* AND **START** *working!*

# I LOVE MYSELF AND DO GOOD THINGS FOR MYSELF!

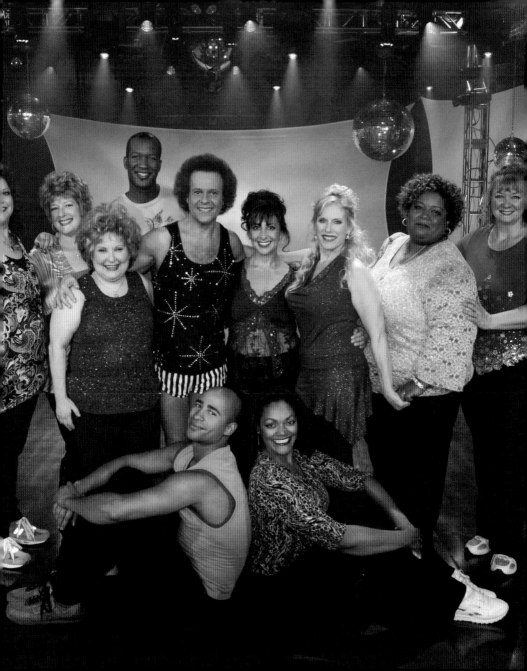

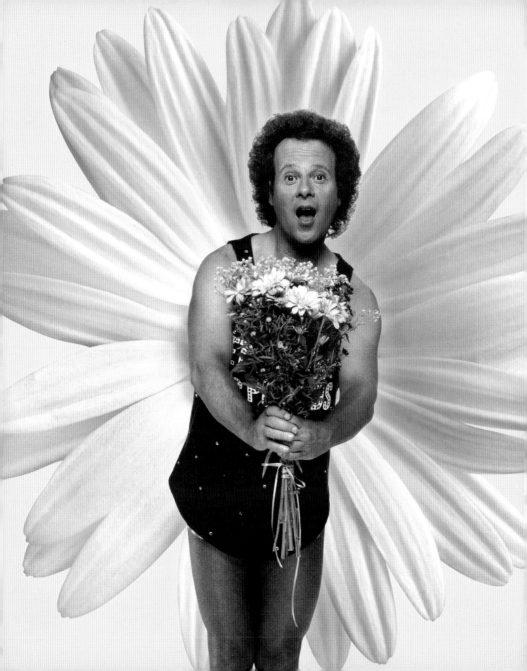

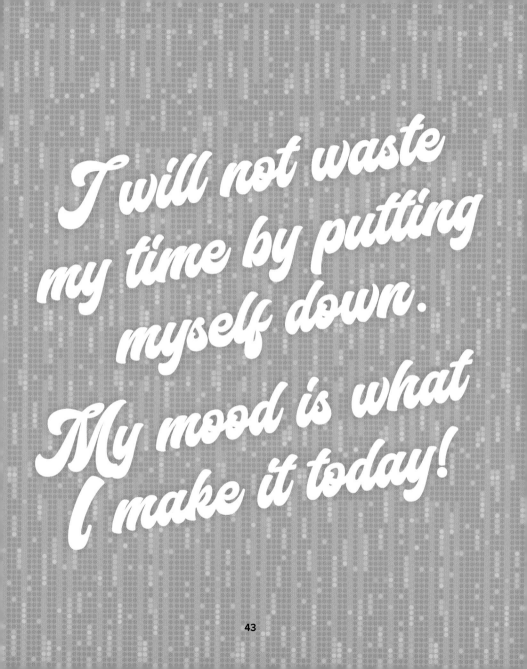

I will not waste my time by putting myself down.

My mood is what I make it today!

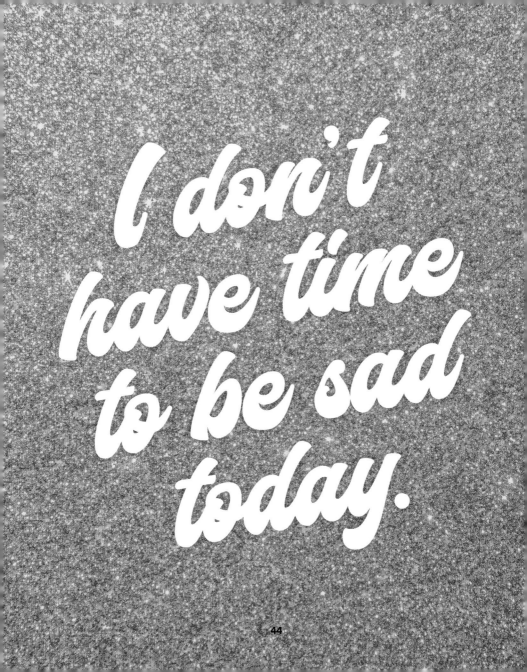

I don't have time to be sad today.

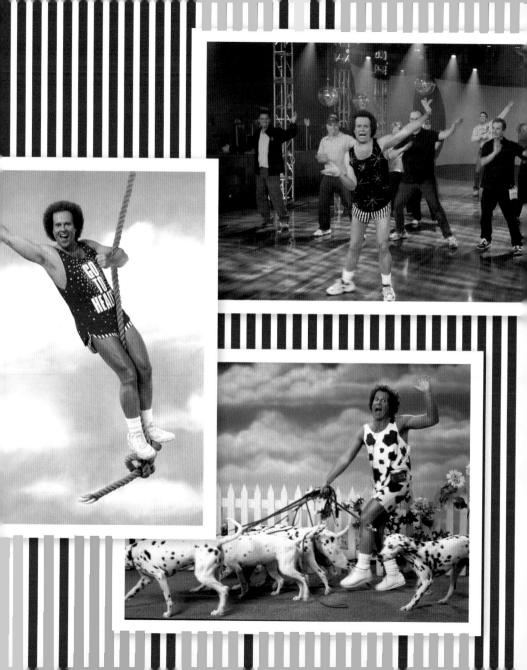

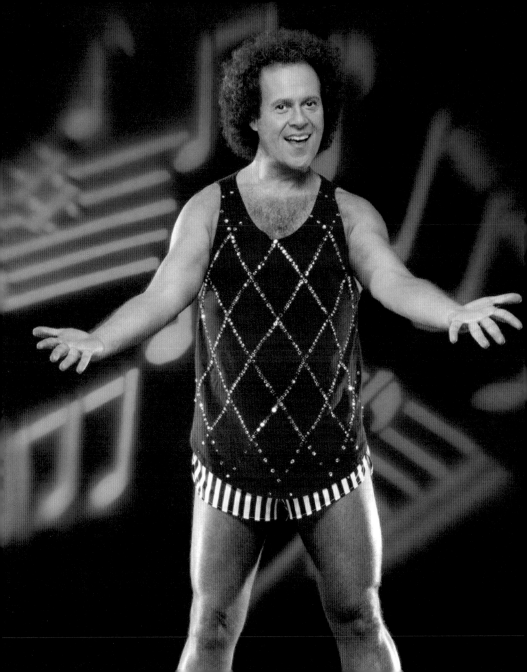

# LIKE A MUSICIAN, I WILL SET THE *rhythm* FOR MY LIFE.

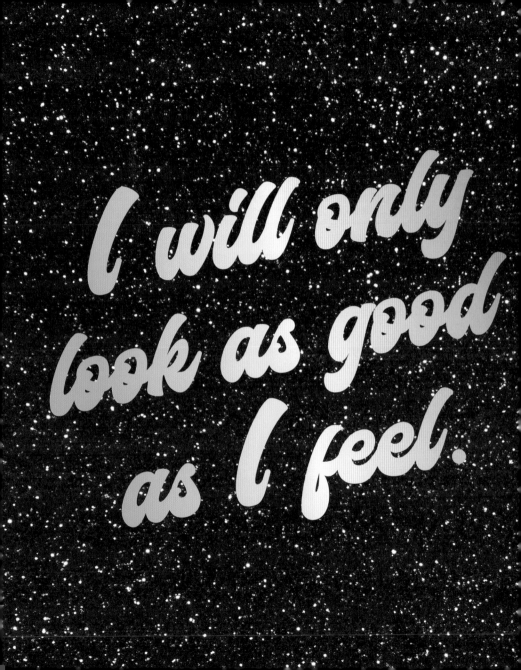

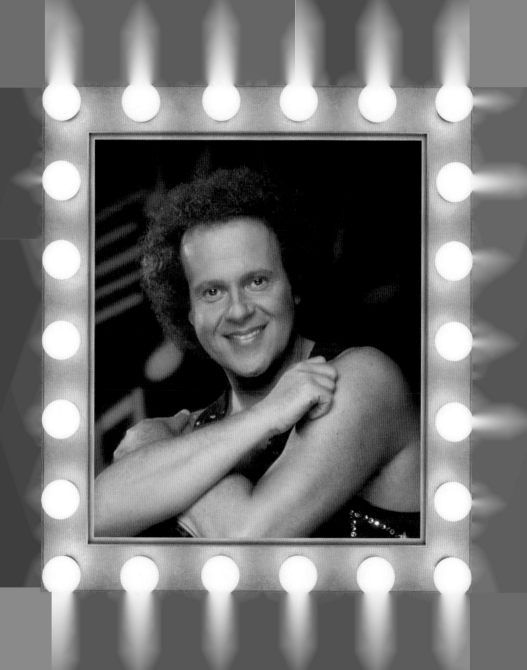

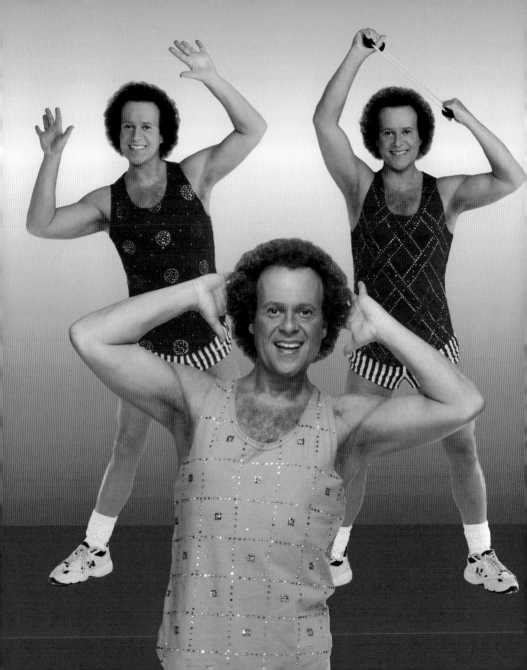

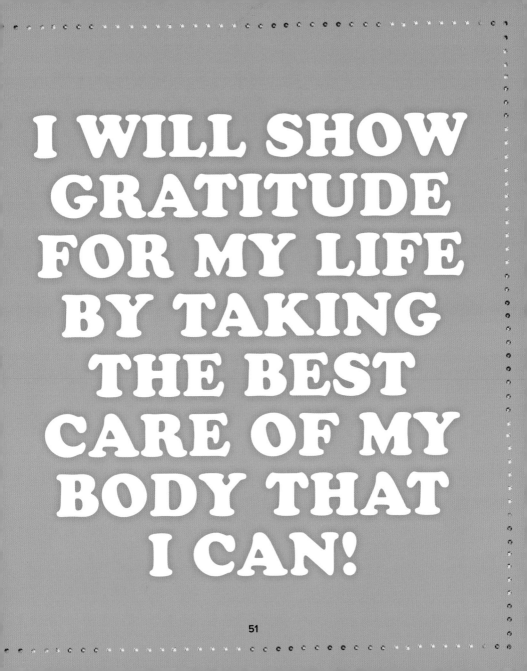

# I WILL SHOW GRATITUDE FOR MY LIFE BY TAKING THE BEST CARE OF MY BODY THAT I CAN!

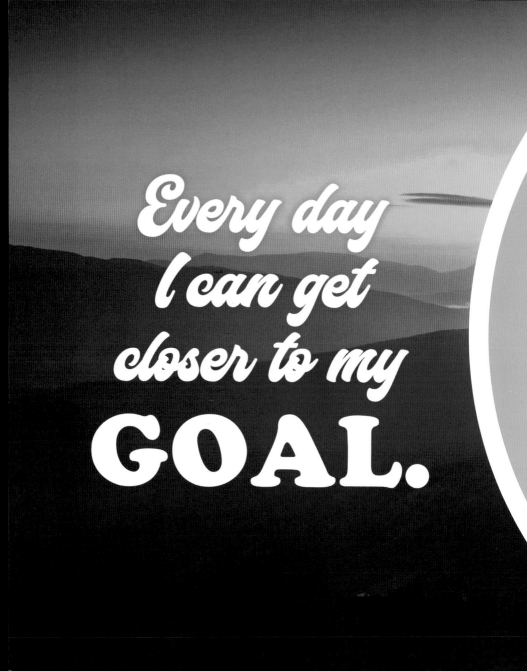

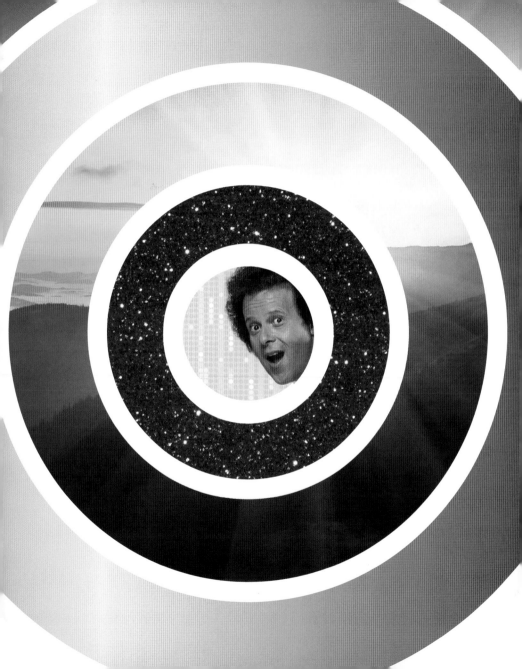

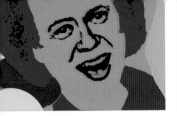
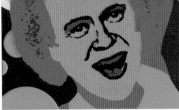
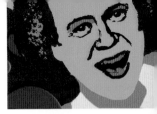
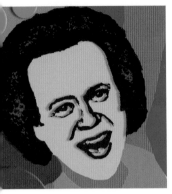
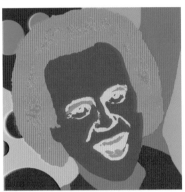
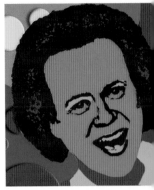
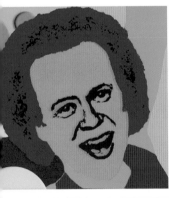
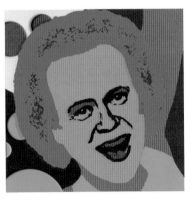
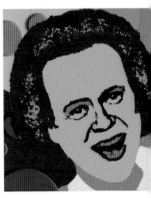
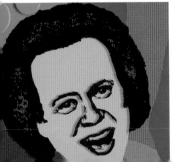
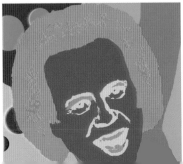
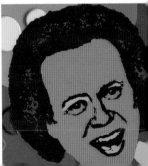

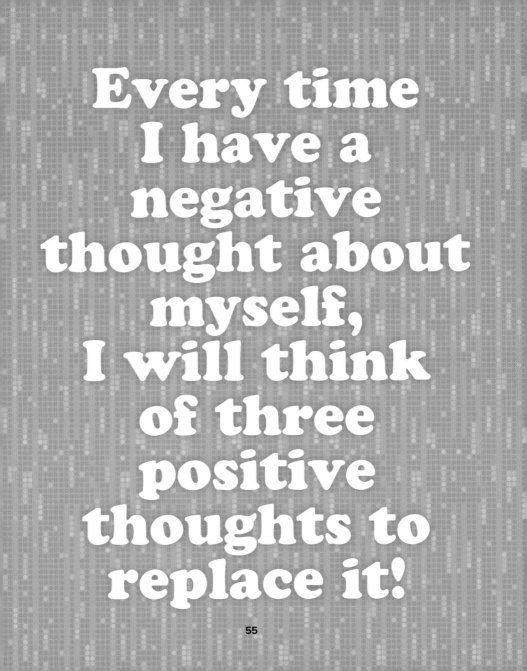

Every time
I have a
negative
thought about
myself,
I will think
of three
positive
thoughts to
replace it!

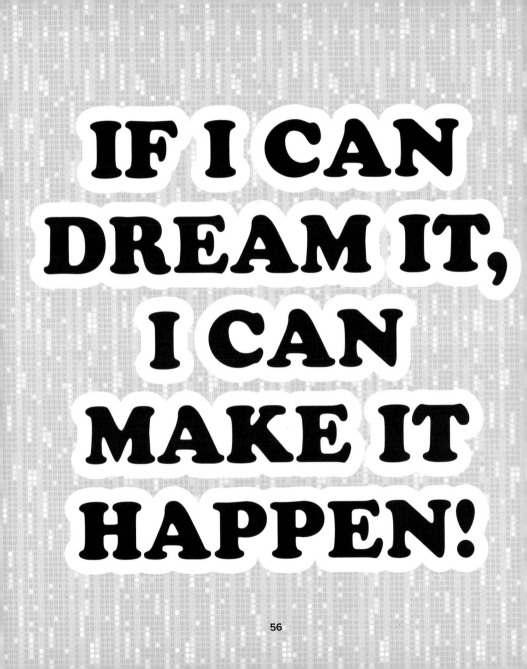

IF I CAN DREAM IT, I CAN MAKE IT HAPPEN!

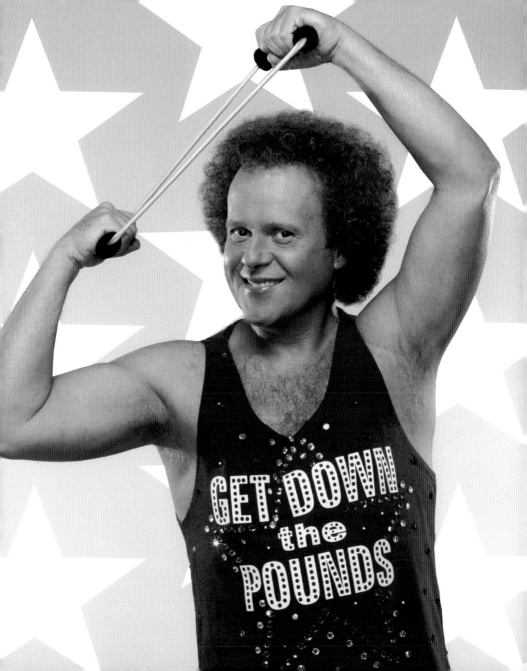

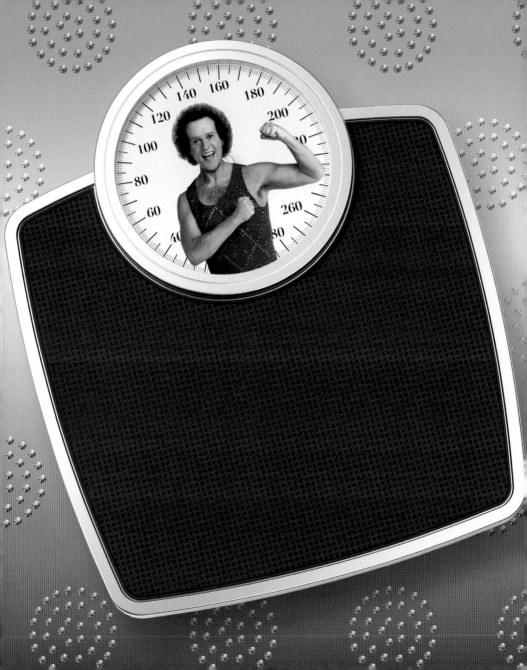

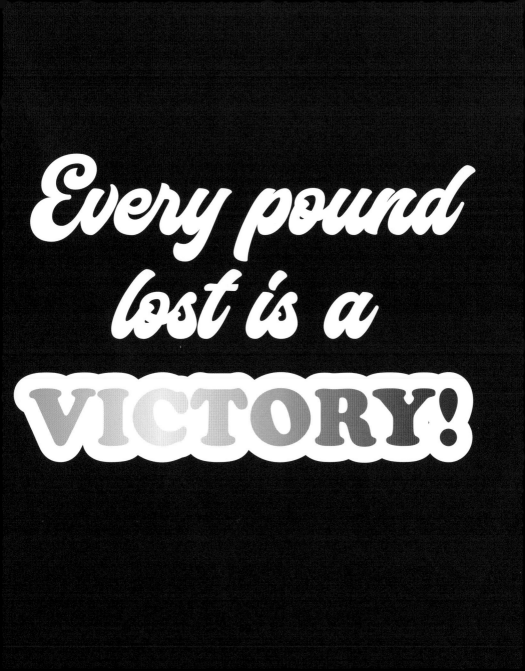

I WILL SET A GOOD EXAMPLE FOR THOSE I LOVE . . . BY TAKING CARE OF ME!

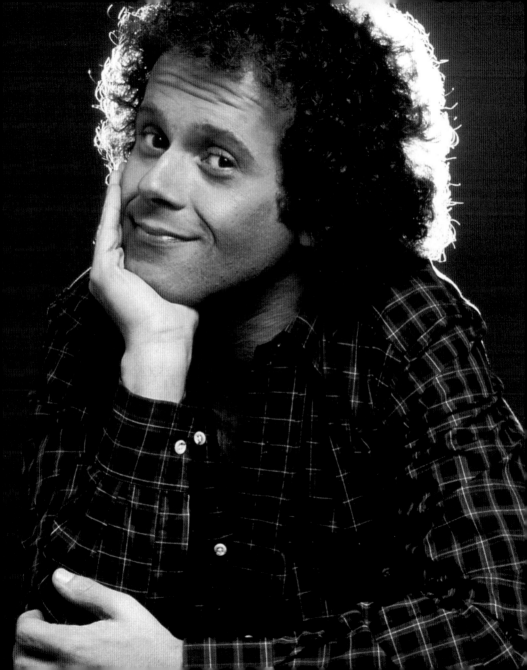

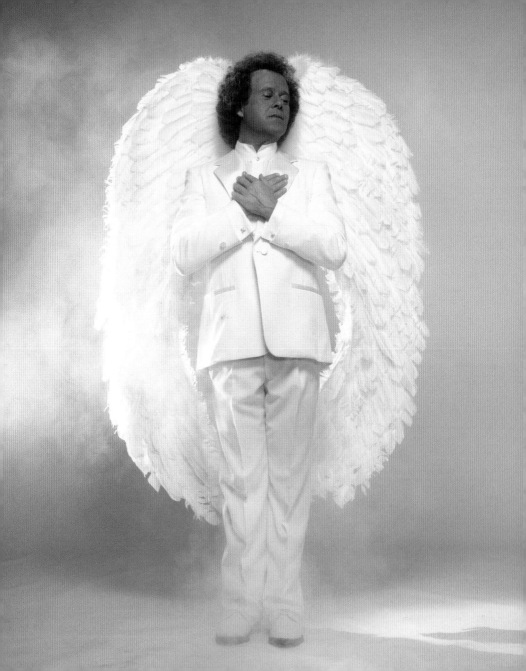

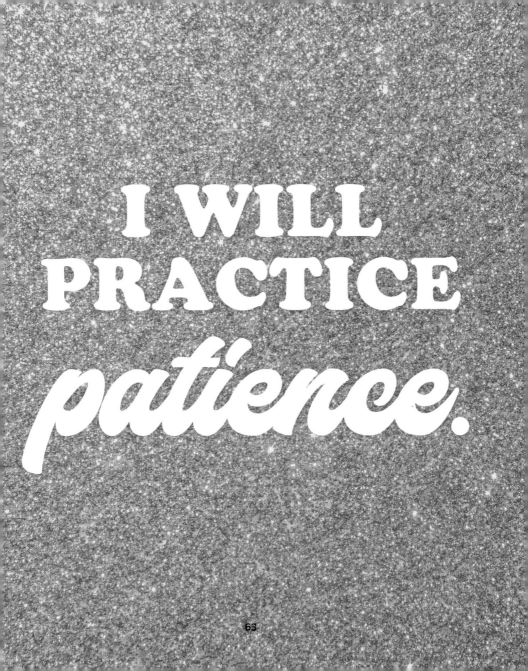

I WILL PRACTICE *patience.*

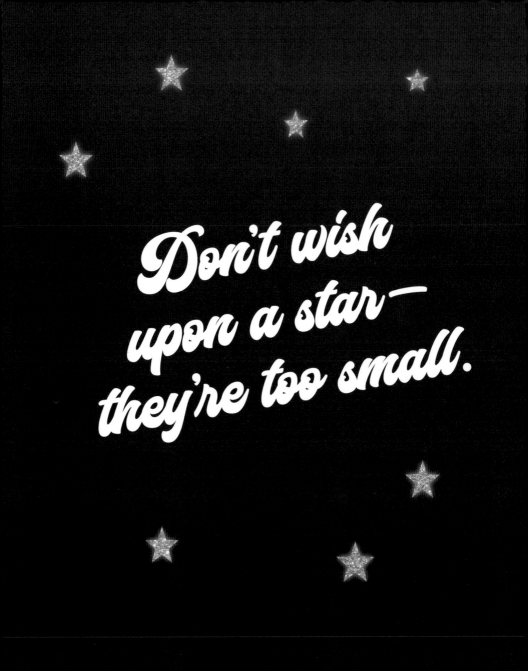

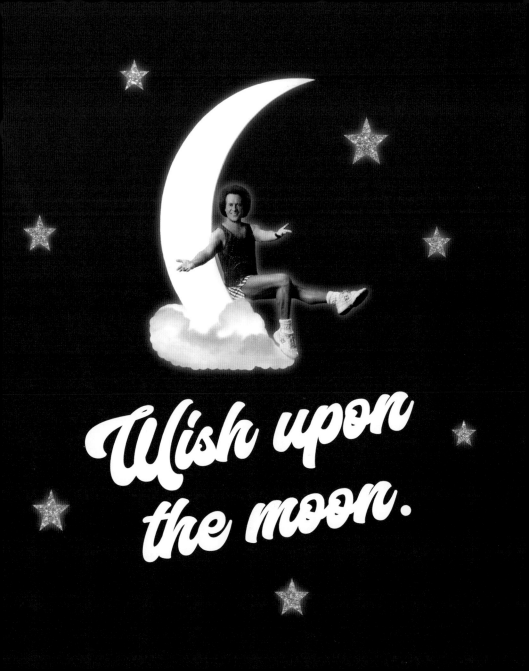

Wish upon the moon.

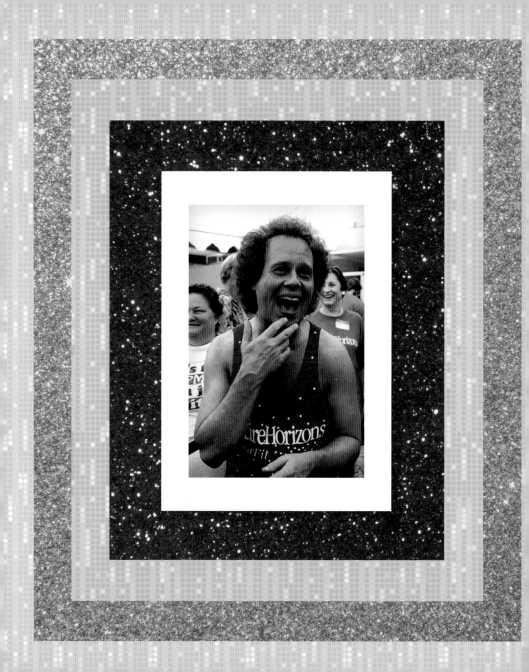

# I AM RESPONSIBLE FOR MY OWN *happiness.*

# A dream is just a dream. A goal is a dream with a plan and a deadline.

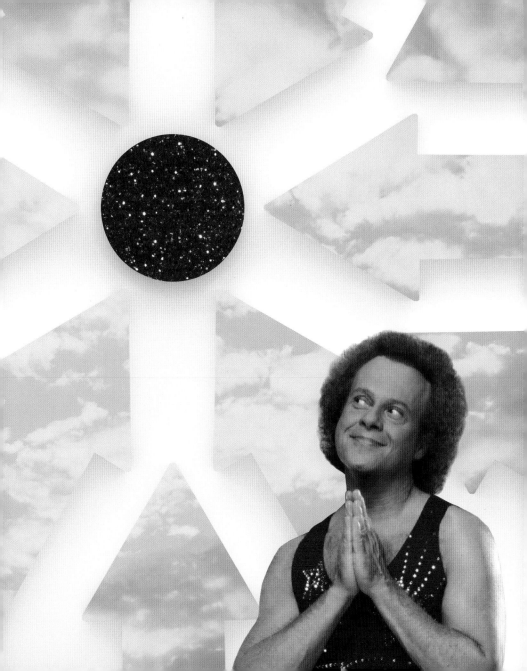

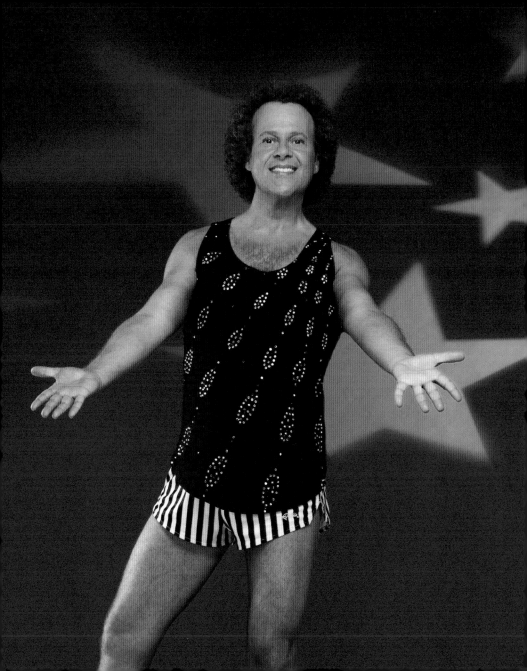

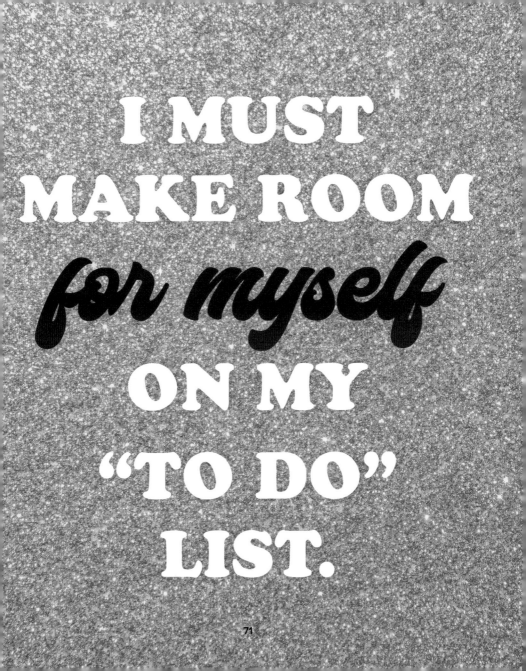

I MUST MAKE ROOM *for myself* ON MY "TO DO" LIST.

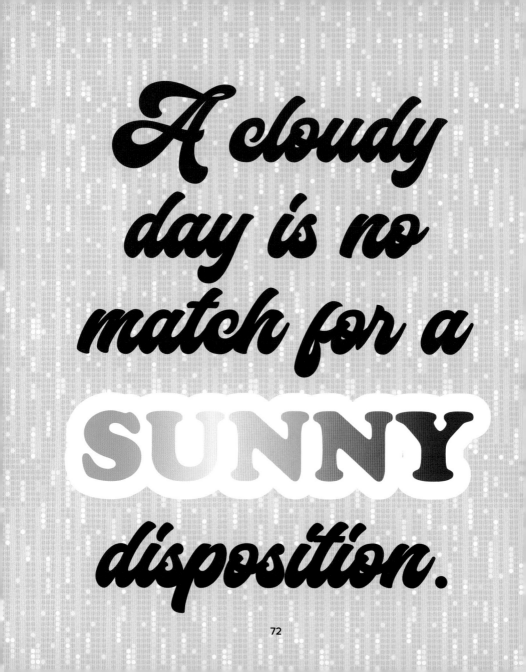

A cloudy day is no match for a SUNNY disposition.

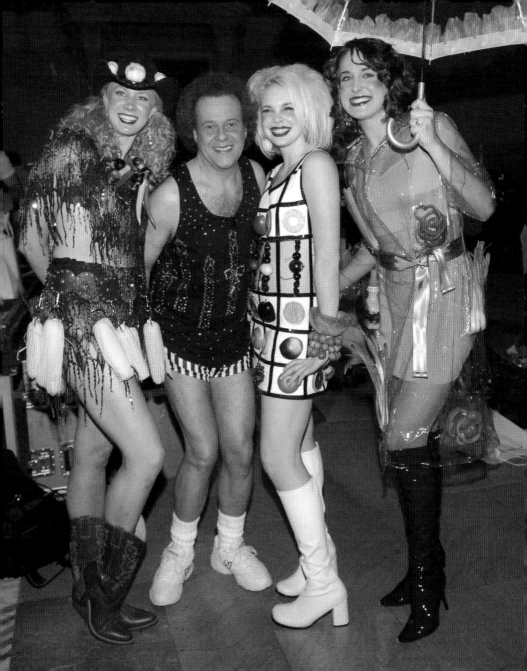

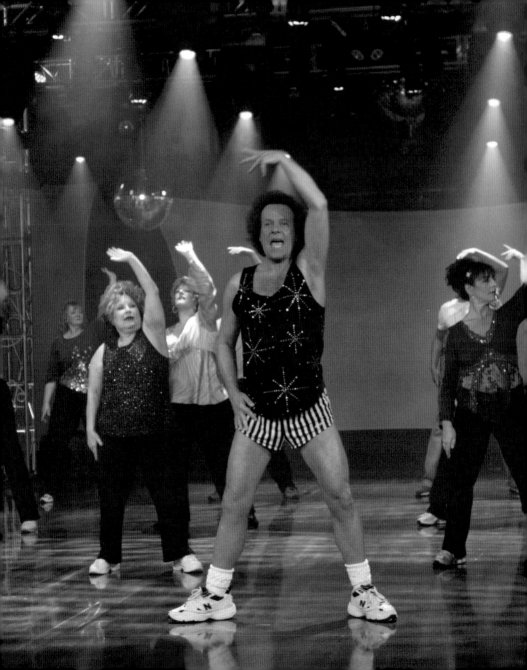

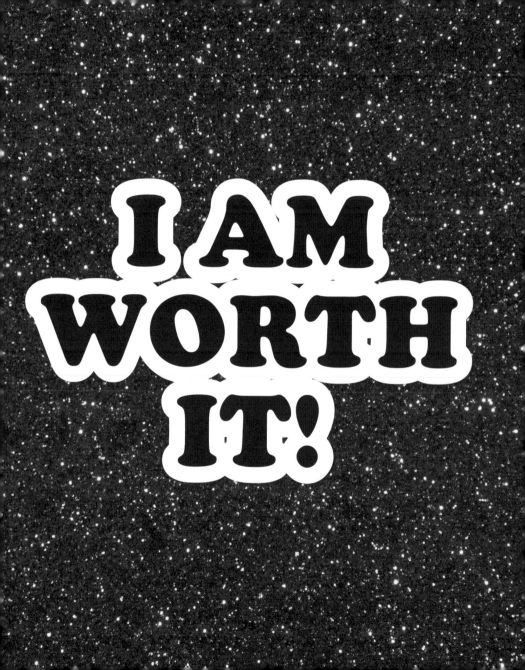

# I will find something to laugh about every day!

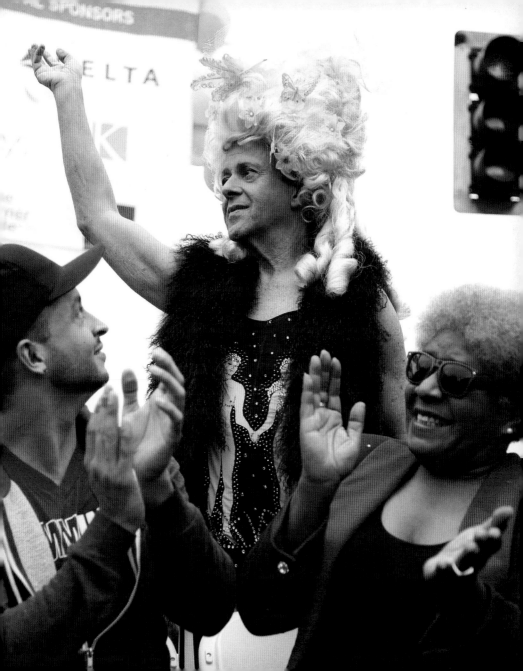

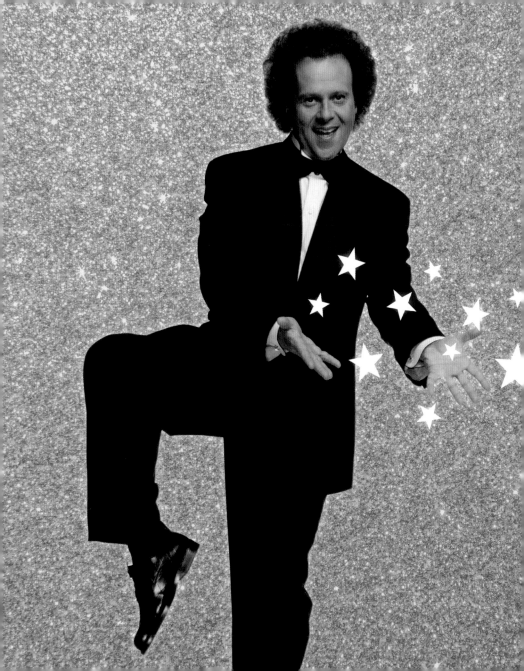

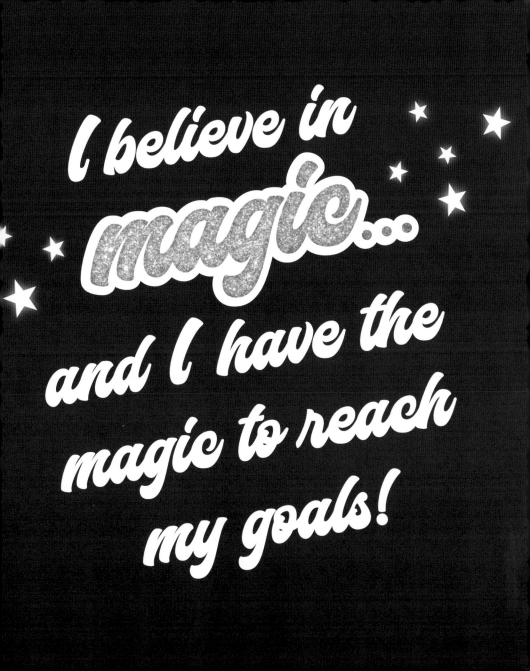

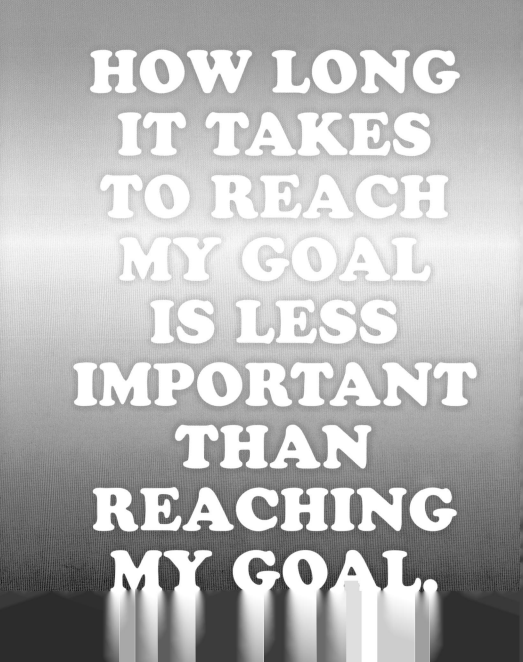

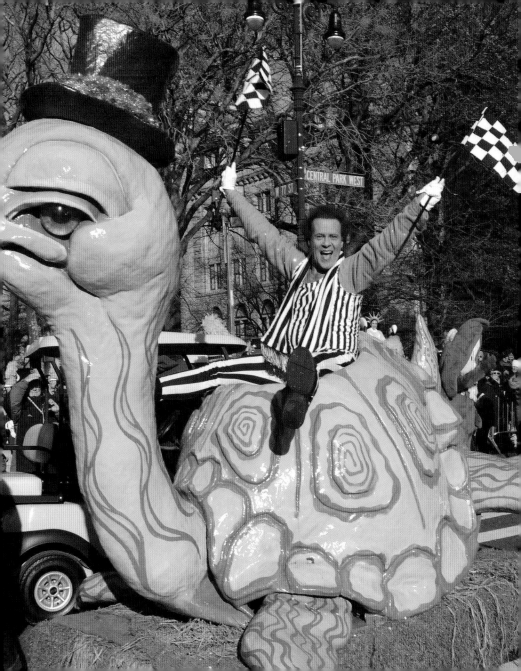

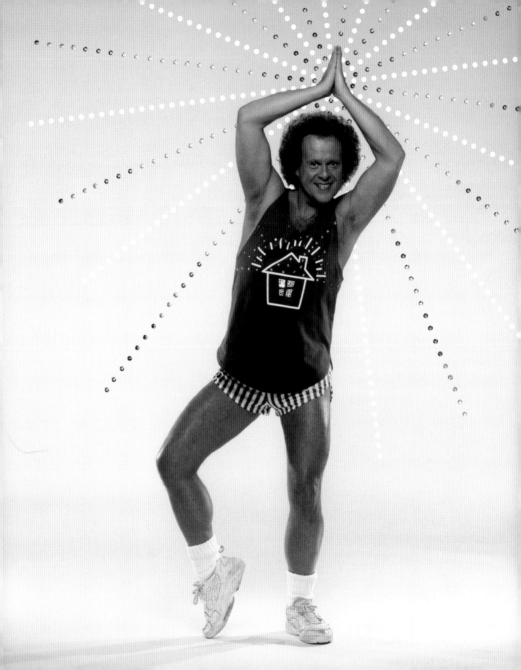

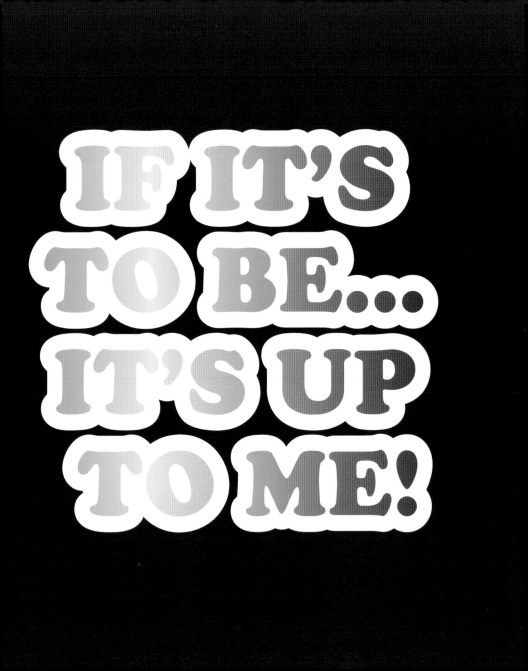

**Repeat after me:**

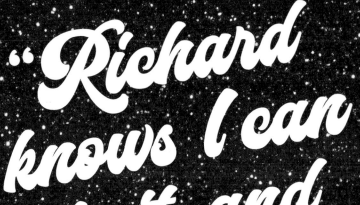
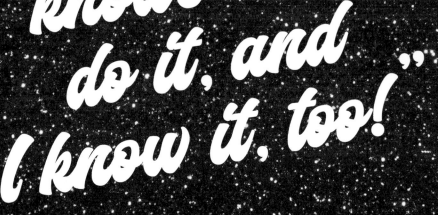

"Richard knows I can do it, and I know it, too!"

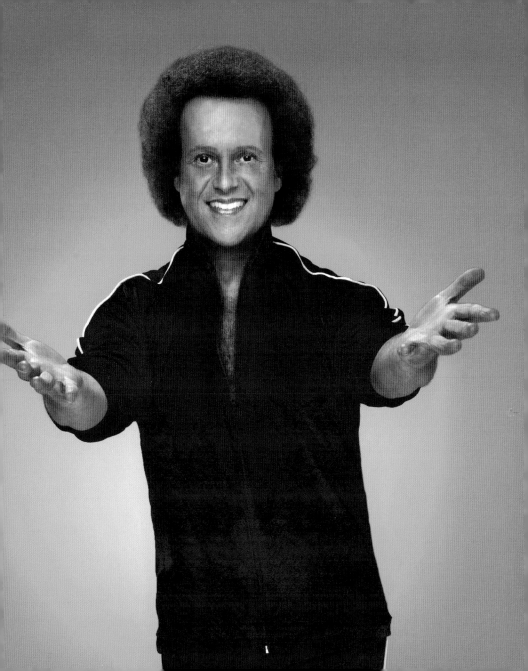

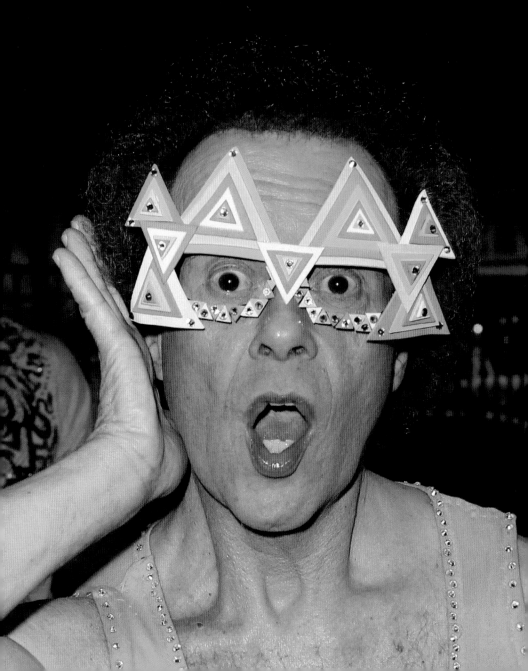

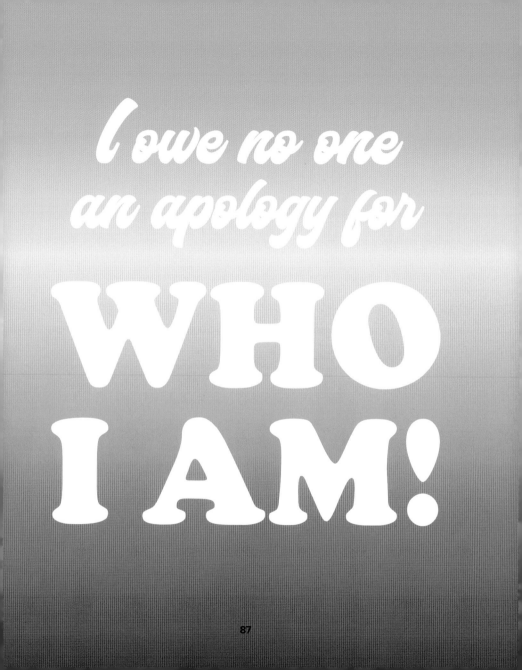

I owe no one an apology for

# WHO I AM!

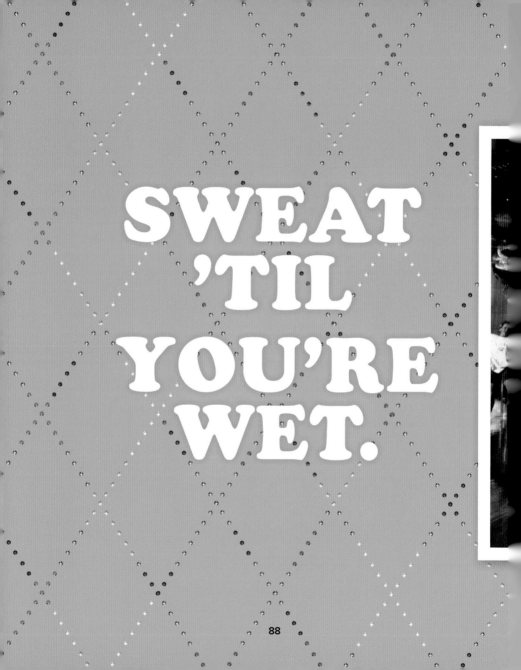

# SWEAT 'TIL YOU'RE WET.

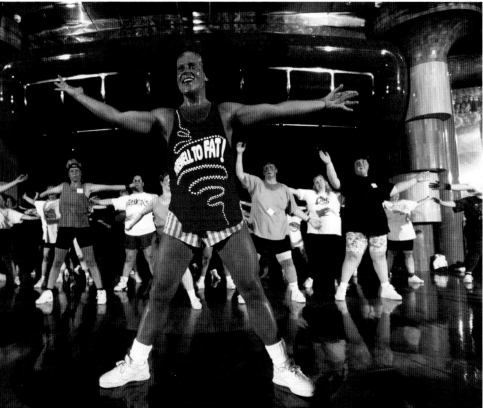

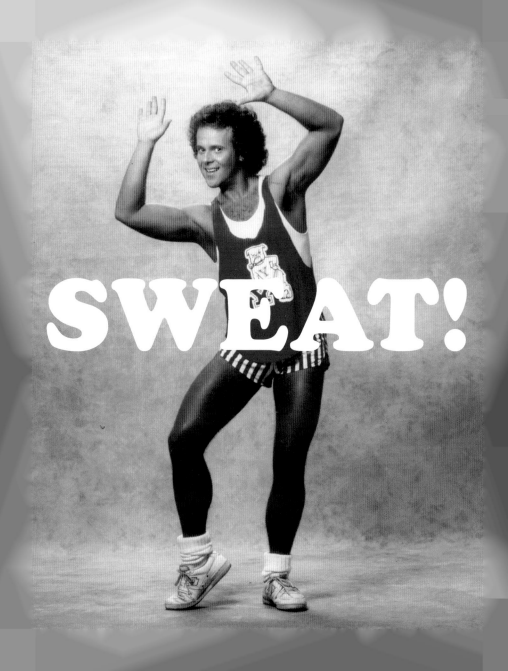

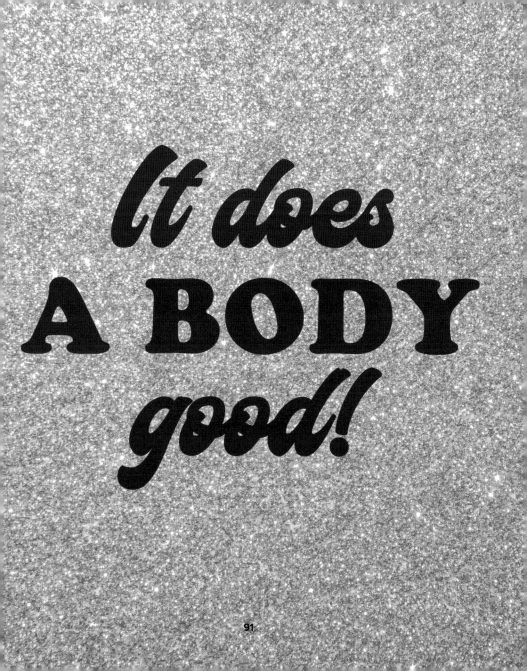

It does
A BODY
good!

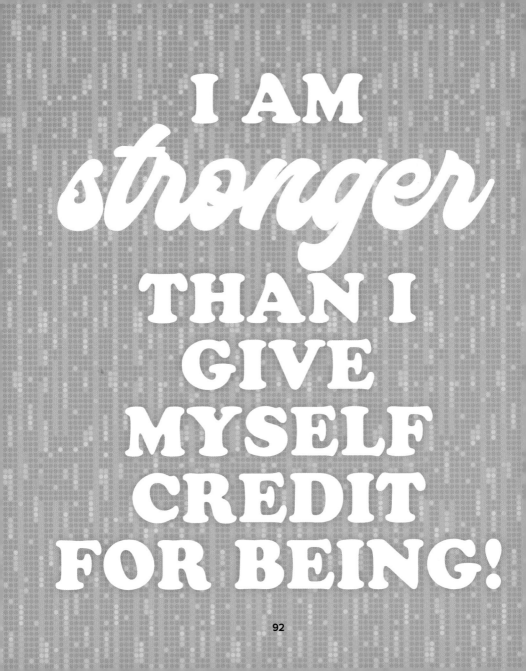

I AM *stronger* THAN I GIVE MYSELF CREDIT FOR BEING!

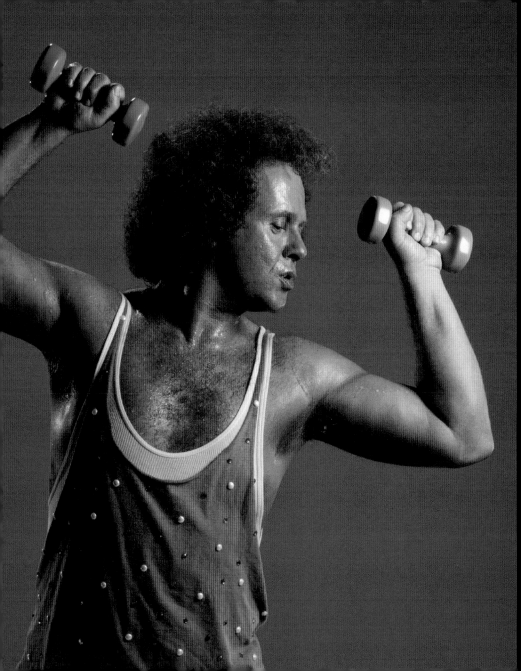

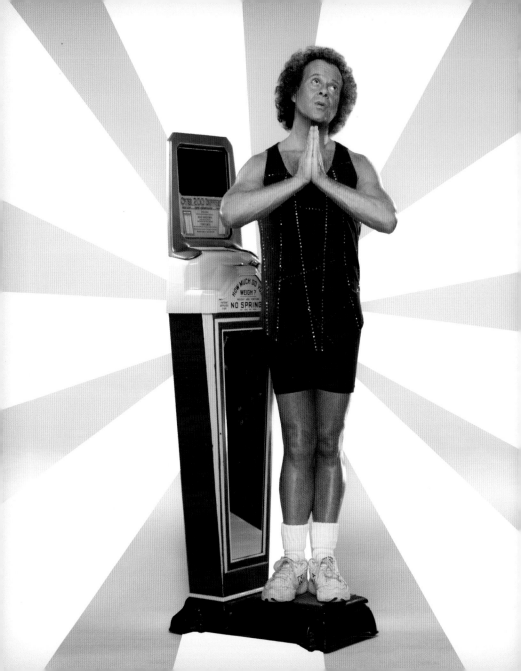

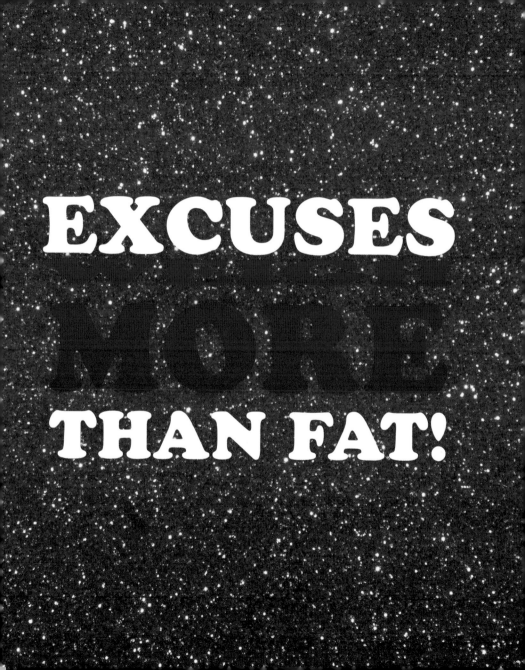

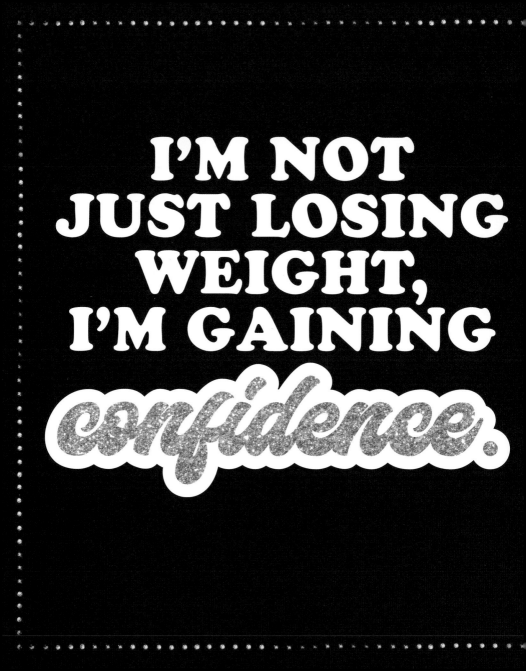

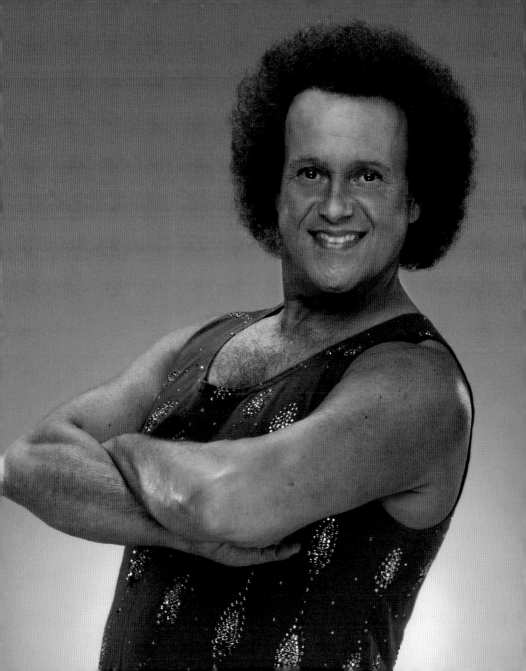

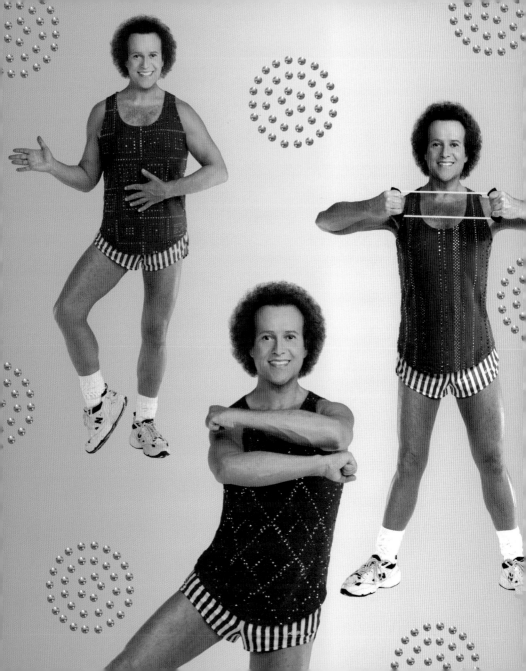

I know that by doing a great workout, I'm doing great things for both my body and my mind.

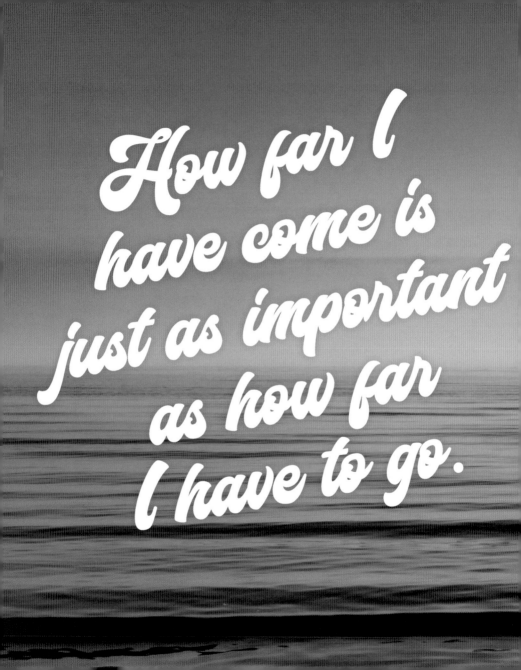

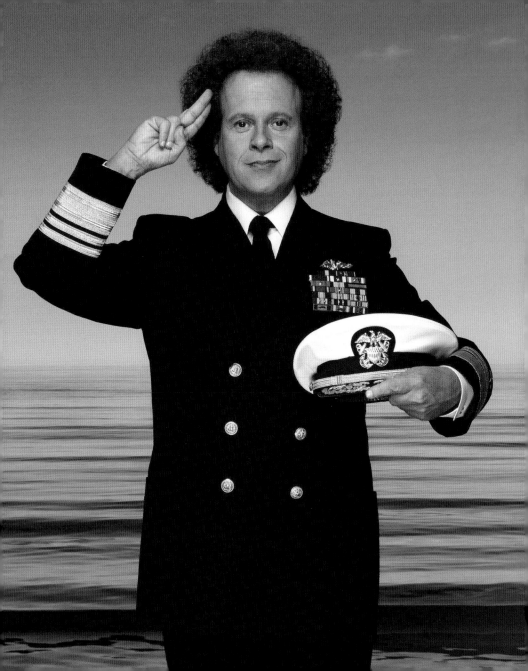

I DON'T FEAR MY FAILURE;

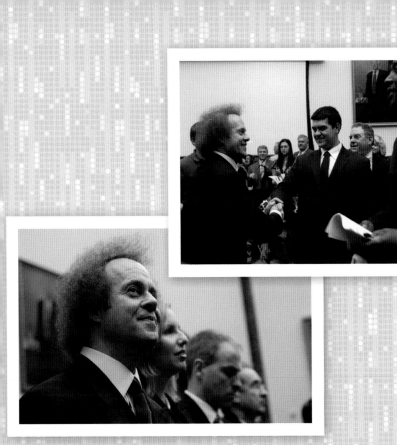

# I'M EXCITED ABOUT MY

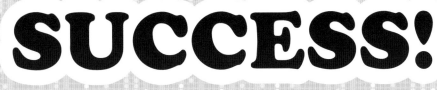

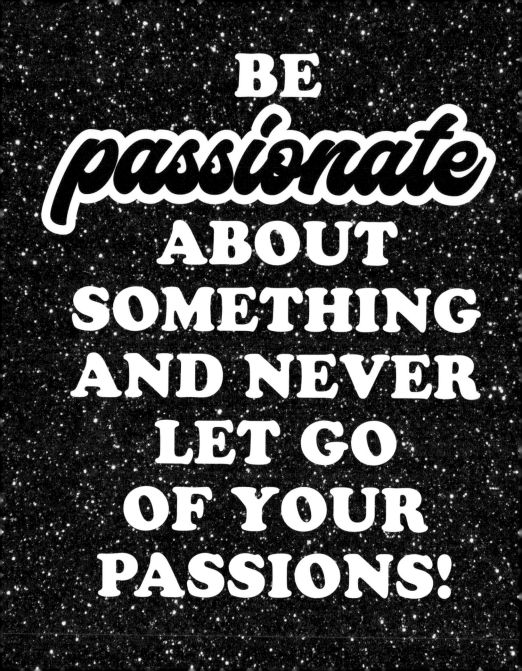

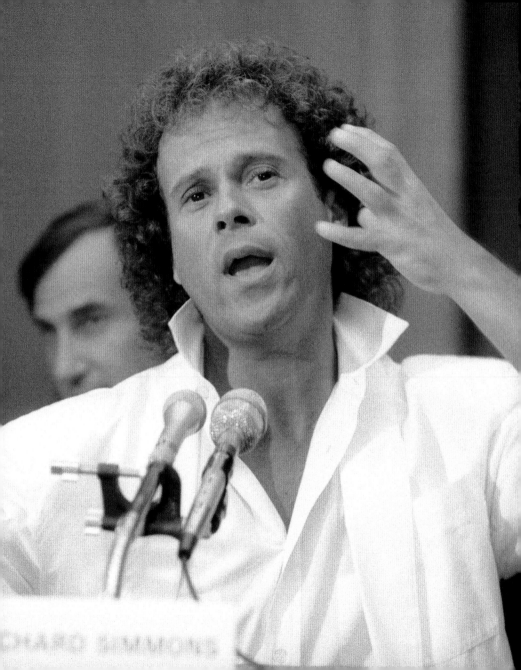

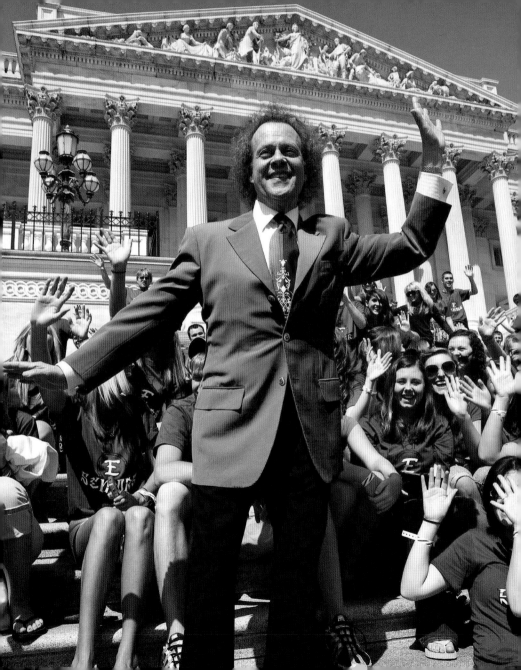

# I will do something today that will make me proud tomorrow!

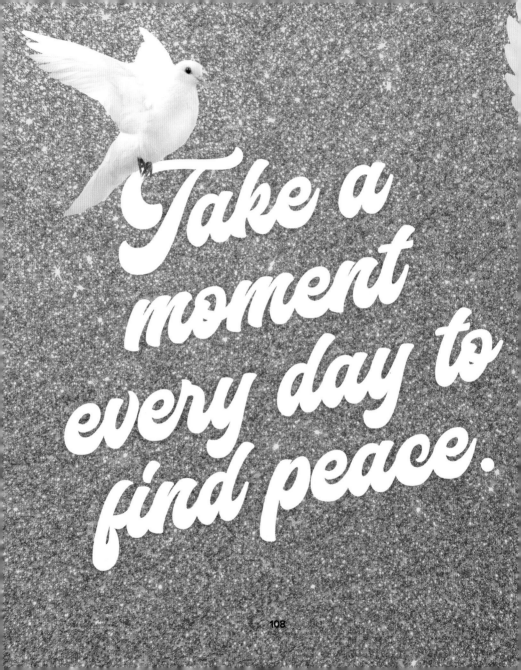

Take a moment every day to find peace.

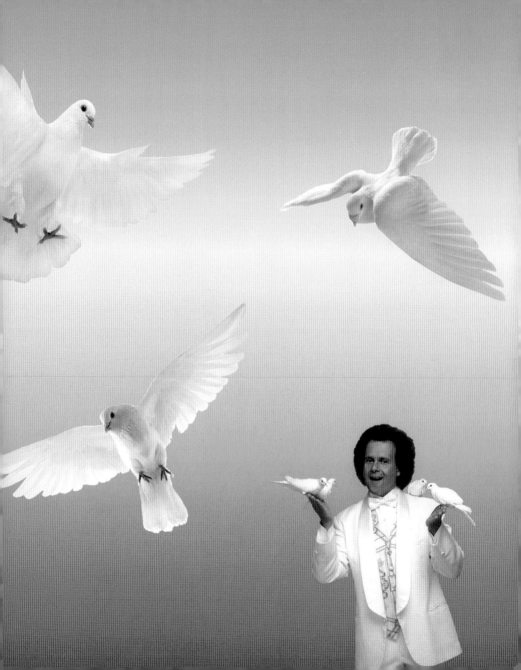

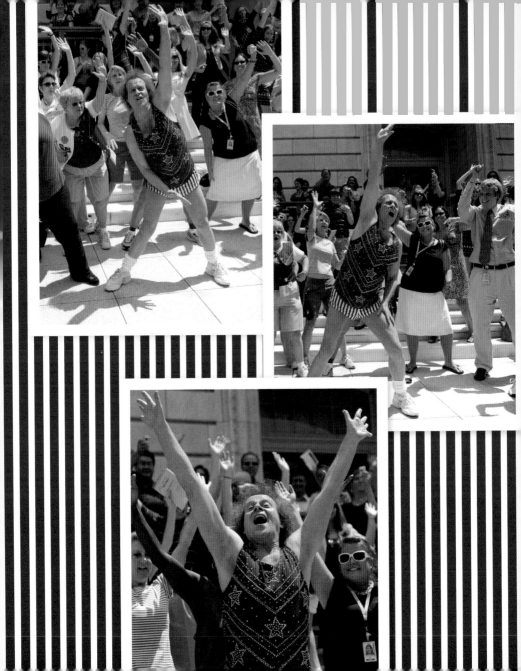

We all have twenty-four hours in our day. It's how we spend those hours that makes the difference!

# Remember, you are one of a kind. There is no one else like you!

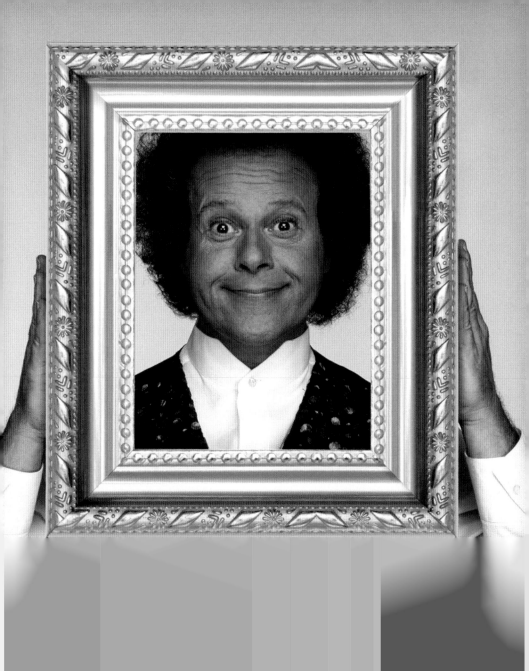

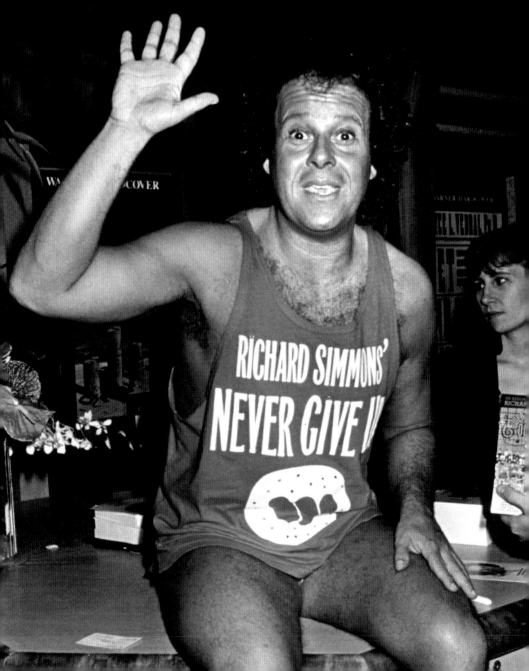

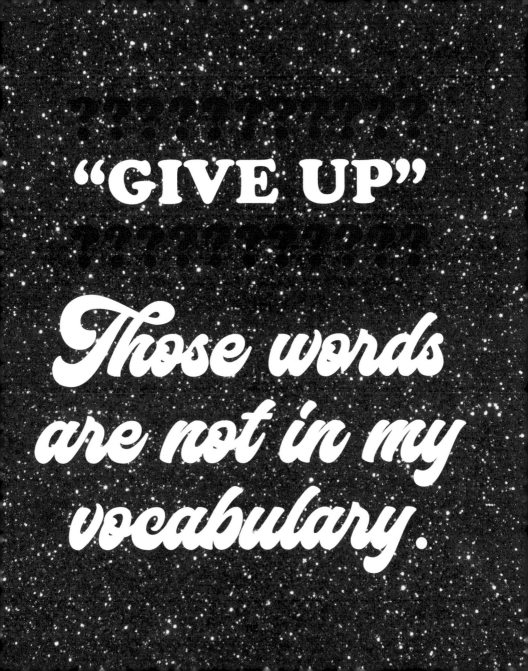

# NO ONE IS PERFECT— ABSOLUTELY NO ONE. LIKE PRECIOUS STONES, WE HAVE A FEW FLAWS.

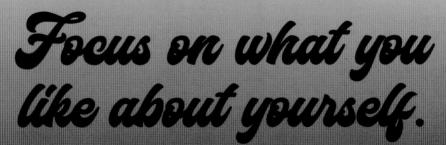

*Focus on what you like about yourself.*

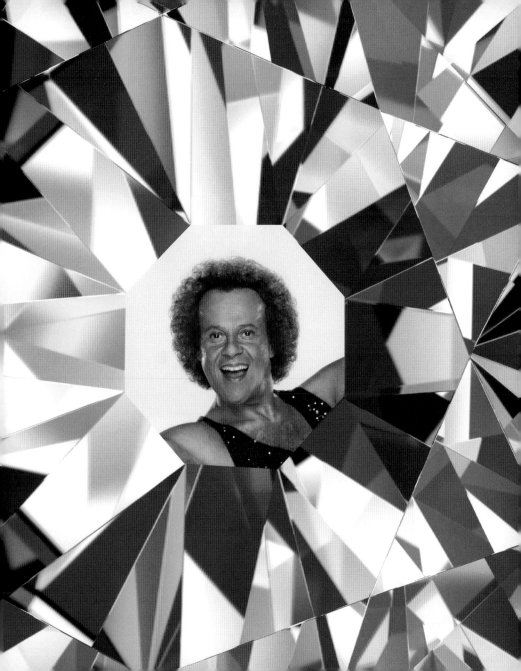

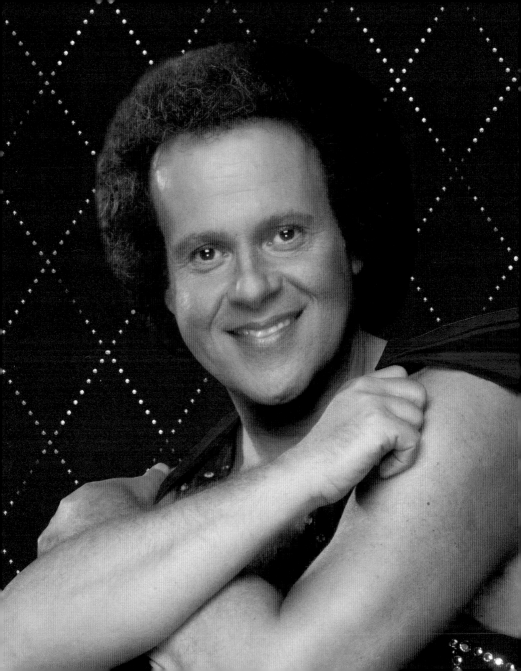

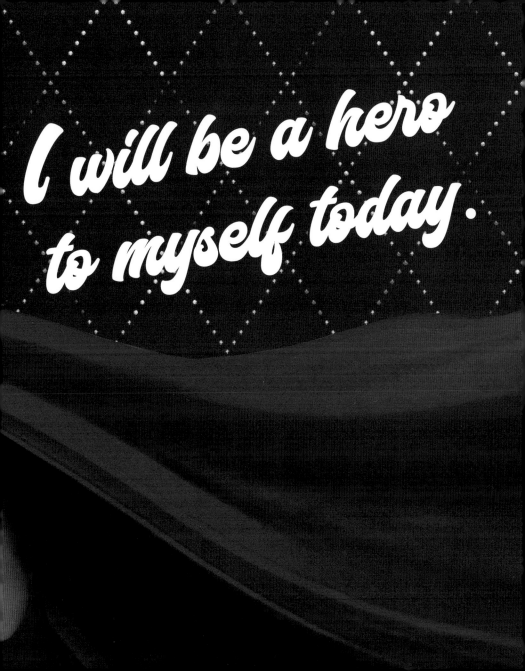

IT'S NEVER TOO LATE TO START AGAIN!

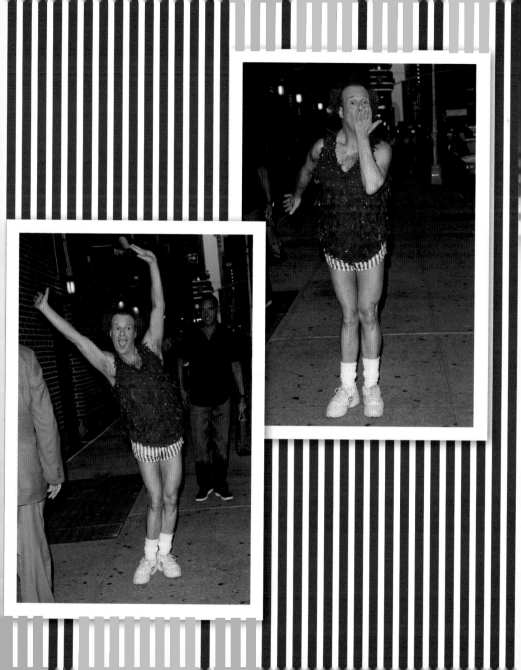

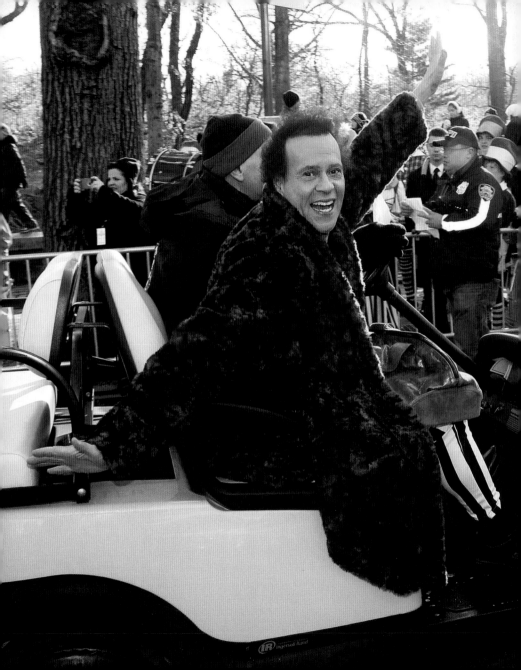